636.1 : 591·4
SOR

·sholt College Library

email library@sparsholt.ac.uk

D1556427

WITHDRAWN

Sparsholt College Library
Sparshott, Winchester
Hants. SO21 2NF

THE

ACC

06 1619 WITHDRAWN

CLASS   636.1; 591.4 SOR

EQUINE THERMOGRAPHY IN PRACTICE

WITHDRAWN

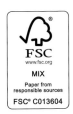

FSC
www.fsc.org
MIX
Paper from
responsible sources
FSC® C013604

EQUINE THERMOGRAPHY IN PRACTICE

Dr Maria Soroko

Department of Horse Breeding and Equestrian Studies, Wroclaw University of Environmental and Life Sciences, Wroclaw, Poland

and

Dr Mina C.G. Davies Morel

Institute of Biological, Environmental and Rural Sciences, Aberystwyth University, Ceredigion, UK

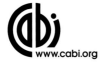

www.cabi.org

CABI is a trading name of CAB International

CABI	CABI
Nosworthy Way	745 Atlantic Avenue
Wallingford	8th Floor
Oxfordshire OX10 8DE	Boston, MA 02111
UK	USA

Tel: +44 (0)1491 832111	
Fax: +44 (0)1491 833508	Tel: +1 (0)617 682 9015
E-mail: info@cabi.org	E-mail: cabi-nao@cabi.org
Website: www.cabi.org	

Originally published in Polish under the title *Termografia Koni w Praktyce* by Stowarzyszenie na Rzecz Zrownowazonego Rozwoju [Association for Sustainable Development], ISBN 978 83 939460 0 6.
© Wroclaw 2014.

© M. Soroko and M.C.G. Davies Morel, 2016. All rights reserved. No part of this publication may be reproduced in any form or by any means, electronically, mechanically, by photocopying, recording or otherwise, without the prior permission of the copyright owners.

A catalogue record for this book is available from the British Library, London, UK.

Library of Congress Control Number: 2016935227

ISBN-13: 978 1 78064 787 6

Commissioning editor: Caroline Makepeace
Associate editor: Alexandra Lainsbury
Production editor: Lauren Povey

Typeset by SPi, Pondicherry, India.
Printed and bound by Replika Press Pvt Ltd, India.

Contents

About the Authors

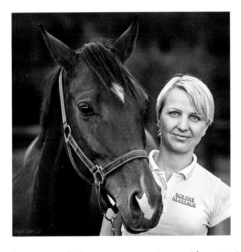

Dr Maria Soroko gained her PhD in Agricultural Science with a specialization in Animal Husbandry from the University of Environmental and Life Sciences of Wroclaw, Department of Horse Breeding and Equestrian Studies in 2013. Her Master's degree in Equine Science was completed in 2010 at the Institute of Biological, Environmental and Rural Sciences, Aberystwyth University, Wales, United Kingdom.

Since 2008, the author has practised thermography extensively in equine physiotherapy and in veterinary medicine, cooperating with veterinarians, horse breeders and trainers. She is also the owner and director of the company Equine Massage (http://www.eqma.pl), which offers equine rehabilitation and thermography services, professional courses and workshops associated with horse rehabilitation, and the application of thermography in veterinary and sports medicine.

Maria conducts research on the application of thermography in sport and racing horses, and has authored numerous original publications and overview papers. She is also a member of the European Association of Thermology.

She has many years of experience in equine physiotherapy, achieving qualifications as an Equine Body Worker in sport massage and remedial therapy. Maria is also a riding instructor at the British Horse Society. Her skills and experience were achieved in both Europe and Australia.

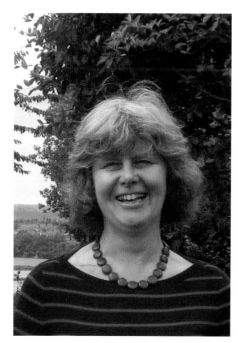

Dr Mina Davies Morel, PhD, Reg. Anim. Sci., SFHEA, is a Reader at Aberystwyth University. After studying for her degree in Animal Science at Nottingham University she went on to study for her PhD at Aberystwyth University and was then awarded the Animal Health Trust Wooldridge farm livestock personal post-doctoral scholarship to continue her research at the University. As a member of staff of the Welsh Agricultural College she set up the Equine Department and courses. Since joining the University, Mina has headed up the equine courses, and over time has developed and managed as well as taught on a wide range of equine science and studies courses, ranging from Foundation degree to MSc. Mina has particular responsibility for postgraduate students and for many years has been Course Director of the MSc Equine Science and MSc Animal Science courses in addition to supervising research students. Mina attained a University teaching excellence award in 2010 and a Higher Education Academy Senior Fellowship Award in 2014, and has taught and held external examiner/adviser positions in numerous universities in the UK and abroad. She has published widely in the scientific and popular press in addition to being the author of three text books. Mina has been a horse owner and rider since childhood.

Acknowledgements

Special thanks go to Maria's uncle, Professor Krzysztof (Kris) Cena, who encouraged her to take a serious interest in research and offered indispensable advice. We would also like to thank Andrzej Soroko for providing the figures and illustrations, and Dr Kevin Howell for reviewing the manuscript.

Maria Soroko
2016

Glossary

General Terms

Body surface temperature: the skin surface temperature, with or without the hair coat.

Cantle: the raised area at the rear of the saddle.

Chronic inflammation: the chronic inflammatory stage, characterized by a prolonged immunological reaction by the body, such as increased body temperature, soreness and/or swelling.

Clinical inflammation: the apparent stage of inflammation, characterized by increased body temperature, pain, lameness and swelling.

Distal forelimbs: the area of the forelimb from the carpal joints to the hooves.

Distal hindlimbs: the area of the hindlimb from the tarsal joints to the hooves.

Equine locomotor system: includes the skeletal system (bones), referred to as the passive locomotor, plus the muscular system, referred to as the active locomotor.

Pommel: the raised area at the front of the saddle.

Subclinical inflammation: a very early stage of inflammation, characterized by the absence of apparent signs of clinical inflammation such as pain, lameness and swelling.

Subluxation: minor dislocation of vertebral joint(s) or a negatively altered relationship between neighbouring vertebra.

Topographical Terms

Back area: includes the thoracic and lumbar vertebrae from the dorsal aspect.

Caudal: structures that lie towards the tail (Fig. G1).

Chest area: includes the thoracic and lumbar vertebrae from the lateral aspect, the chest and part of the flank area.

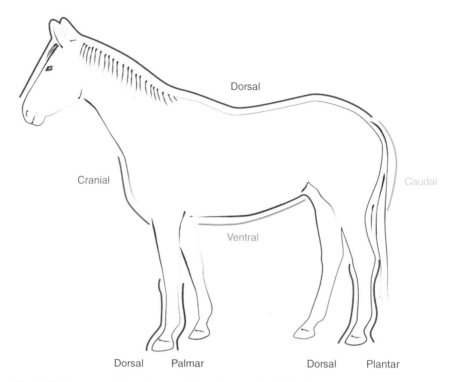

Fig. G1. Topographical terms: lateral aspect of the horse.

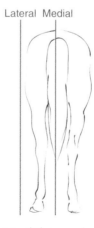

Fig. G2. Topographical terms: caudal aspect of the horse.

Cranial: structures that lie towards the chest (Fig. G1).
Croup area: includes the sacral and coccygeal vertebrae, tuber coxae, gluteus muscles, hip joint, tuber ischii, femur, patella, stifle joint, gaskin and part of the flank area (depending on the projection).

Dorsal: structures that lie towards the head, neck, back and croup; structures of the distal forelimbs and hindlimbs that lie towards the cranial end (Fig. G1).

Lateral: structures that lie towards the side of the animal (Fig. G2).

Medial: structures that lie towards the median plane that divides the body into two symmetrical (right and left) halves (Fig. G2).

Neck area: includes the dorsal, lateral and ventral aspects of the neck plus the jugular vein.

Palmar: structures of the distal forelimbs that lie towards the caudal end (Fig. G1).

Plantar: structures of the distal hindlimbs that lie towards the caudal end (Fig. G1).

Shoulder area: includes the withers, scapula, shoulder joint, triceps brachii muscle, humerus and elbow joint.

Ventral: structures that lie towards the abdomen (Fig. G1).

Introduction

Equine Thermography in Practice is a compendium of the practical application of thermography to equine veterinary medicine and rehabilitation. Currently, thermography is one of the most rapidly evolving equine diagnostic tools. Intensive training of horses is associated with significant physical demands on the musculoskeletal system, contributing to a high incidence of injury. Injury causes changes in blood circulation and thereby changes in body surface temperature. Thermography can detect these changes in body surface temperature and hence can be used to diagnose and monitor injury, disease and work overload of the musculoskeletal system.

This book aims to provide a valuable source of reference for equine thermographers, veterinarians, equine therapists and body manipulators, as well as farriers, equine podiatrists, saddlers, riders, trainers and other paraprofessionals in the equine industry. As a reference text book, it will also prove useful to students of veterinary medicine, animal/equine science and husbandry, as well as students of other courses where equine science is studied.

This book is the first publication on the equestrian book market that extensively discusses equine thermography issues and its use in equine diagnosis.

If you have any comments, suggestions or queries concerning this book, please contact Maria Soroko by email at kontakt@eqma.pl, and also on www.facebook.com/EquineThermographyPractice. Any feedback is very much appreciated.

1 Principles of Equine Thermography

1.1 Thermography

Thermography is a non-invasive diagnostic method, based on body surface temperature detection. The infrared radiation emitted from the body surface is recorded and visualized in the form of a temperature distribution map. The resulting 'thermogram' can be used to determine physiological changes to, and reflect blood flow patterns and the speed of metabolism in, the body of a horse (Turner, 1991). It also reflects the impact of environmental factors during examination.

> In order to obtain reliable thermographic measurements of the horse's body surface temperature, the examination should be carried out on a carefully prepared animal and in an appropriate examination room.

Constant body temperature is a characteristic feature among warm-blooded animals. During exercise, working muscles produce substantial quantities of heat, which must be eliminated from the body in order to prevent the animal from overheating. This loss of heat is achieved through sweating (evaporation), heat conduction, air flow (convection) and infrared radiation. In cold weather conditions, the animal starts thermogenesis (heat production) in order to maintain a constant body temperature (Ivanov, 2006). The skin and hair coat play an important role in the process of heat exchange between the body and the environment. Skin also acts as a thermal perception organ, informing the animal about environmental conditions, including changes in temperature and humidity. Hence, the body surface temperature of a horse as measured by thermography is the combined result of the heat produced by the body and the impact of environmental factors.

© M. Soroko and M.C.G. Davies Morel 2016. *Equine Thermography in Practice* (M. Soroko and M.C.G. Davies Morel)

1.2   Methods for Measuring Infrared Radiation

Heat exchange between the body surface and environment by infrared radiation plays a major role in the heat balance of the animal (Cena, 1974). Loss of heat by radiation will take place only when there is a temperature difference between the surface of the animal and the environment. The energy transferred from the body surface by infrared radiation depends on both the physiological processes occurring within the body and the environmental conditions, which in turn influence blood circulation under the skin. Infrared radiation measurement is useful therefore in monitoring physiological changes in animals that result in heat production such as exercise, injury, illness and environmental impact (Purohit and McCoy, 1980; Palmer, 1983; Turner *et al.*, 2001; Soroko *et al.*, 2014).

Infrared radiation can be measured using either a simple pyrometer or a thermographic camera. A pyrometer measures infrared radiation energy from a specific area of the body surface, which is presented as an average temperature value (Fig. 1.1). A thermographic camera, however, produces an image (thermogram) illustrating a map of the radiation energy over a selected body surface area (Fig. 1.2).

1.3   Principles of Infrared Radiation

The origins of thermography can be traced back to the discovery of infrared radiation by the English astronomer Friedrich Wilhelm Herschel in 1800. Infrared

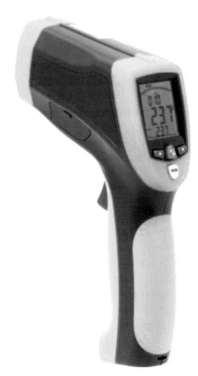

Fig. 1.1. A pyrometer, used for measuring temperature values for a specific area.

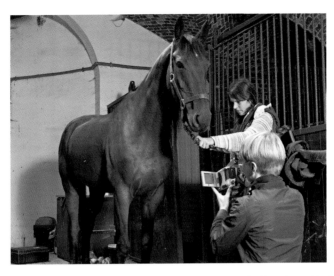

Fig. 1.2. An example of the thermographic measurement with a hand held camera.

radiation is the result of the movement of electrons, and is transmitted from the body surface as electromagnetic waves of varying wavelengths, ranging from 0.7 to 1000 μm (Fig. 1.3). Electromagnetic waves are produced across a spectrum of wavelengths, each wavelength representing a specific type of energy, such as X-rays, ultraviolet light, etc. (Fig. 1.3). A thermal camera measures energy in a specific part of the infrared waveband and correlates this with body surface temperature to produce a colour image illustrating the appropriate temperature values. In this way, body surface temperature is determined without physical contact with the examined animal (Kastberger and Stachl, 2003).

Part of the infrared band of the electromagnetic spectrum is absorbed into the atmosphere, which is why thermal equipment manufacturers produce thermographic cameras with only two types of sensor: short wave and long wave. Short-wave cameras typically detect radiation with wavelengths of 3–5 μm, whereas long-wave cameras are sensitive to wavelengths of 7–14 μm. According to Wien's law (Kastberger and Stachl, 2003), an object with a high surface temperature emits peak radiation at short wavelengths (0.9–5 μm), whereas an object with a lower surface temperature emits peak radiation of long wavelengths (7–14 μm). Therefore, short-wave cameras are designed mostly for industrial use, where high temperature values are recorded, whereas long-wave cameras are used to read lower temperature values, e.g. in the civil engineering sector.

The animal body emits infrared radiation of wavelengths from around 3 to 50 μm. The peak emitted wavelength depends on the ambient temperature. This is related to the following rule: the higher the ambient temperature, the higher the body surface temperature, which results in radiation of shorter wavelengths being emitted. In the case of low ambient temperatures, the lower body surface temperature results in longer-wavelength radiation being emitted (Fig. 1.4). Due to the ambient temperature range typically encountered, long-wave thermal cameras are preferred for animal examinations.

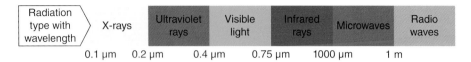

Fig. 1.3. The electromagnetic spectrum, with infrared radiation.

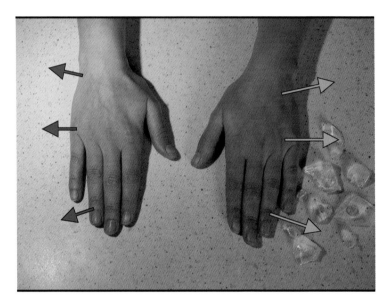

Fig. 1.4. The warm right hand emits short-wave infrared radiation, while the cold left hand emits long-wave infrared radiation.

The body surface of an animal emits infrared electromagnetic waves, thus losing heat, but at the same time it also absorbs heat due to infrared radiation emitted or reflected from other sources, such as other animals, walls and the ground (Fig. 1.5). This can have a significant impact on the recorded body surface temperature (Cena, 1974). The ability of the body to absorb and reflect infrared radiation from other heat sources is a major reason for interference in body surface temperature measurements when examining animals and must be borne in mind when using thermography.

The emitted as well as the absorbed and reflected infrared radiation propagates isotropically (in all directions) from the entire body surface of the animal (Fig. 1.6).

1.4   The Thermographic Image

The measurement of electromagnetic wave energy emitted by the body using a thermal camera enables the creation of a thermographic image (thermogram). A thermogram is created by converting infrared radiation into electrical signals,

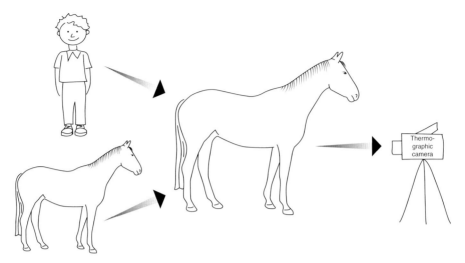

Fig. 1.5. The body surface of the horse emits infrared radiation, and also absorbs and reflects it from surrounding objects.

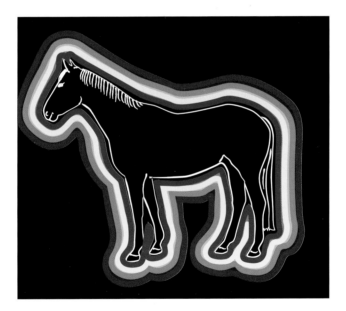

Fig. 1.6. Isotropic emission of infrared radiation from a horse's body surface.

which are then changed into visible-light radiation. This forms an image in a colour palette, in which various colours represent the relevant temperature range. This creates a graphical temperature distribution map of the examined body surface area. The colour bar appearing on the side of the thermogram maps each colour to a temperature range.

Thermograms presented in a simple 'rainbow' palette illustrate the warmest parts of the body in white and red, cooler areas in green and yellow, and the coolest parts in blue and black (Fig. 1.7). The thermograms in this book will be presented in this palette.

An accurate measurement of an animal's body surface temperature is dependent on the determination of the emissivity of the body surface. Emissivity is a measure of the efficiency of the emission of infrared radiation by any given body. Its value can range from 0 to 1, and depends on the emitting surface structure. Emissivity is low in the case of smooth surfaces but high for porous surfaces with a complex structure, such as skin (depending on the skin thickness and hair length). Biological tissues have emissivity values in the range of 0.95–0.98. To obtain the correct manual emissivity setting for a thermal camera, the following steps are carried out:

- Measure the temperature value of a given body area of the animal with a contact thermometer.
- Adjust the temperature reading on the display of the camera to the temperature reading on the contact thermometer.

In practice, emissivity is usually assumed to be 1, which will have a minimal impact on temperature accuracy.

1.5   Thermographic Imaging Technology

Thermographic camera technology has advanced rapidly in recent years, and a number of manufacturers now offer feature-rich infrared imagers at reasonable costs, particularly of the 'uncooled microbolometer' detector type. For equine thermography, a thermal camera should be portable and rugged, as it will be used in demanding outdoor environments. The imager should have a high spatial resolution for maximum image detail, as large-animal thermography is often performed at distances of several metres from the subject. An affordable entry-level imager may have a detector pixel array size of 320 × 240 elements. Superior image detail can be obtained with 640 × 480 pixel arrays,

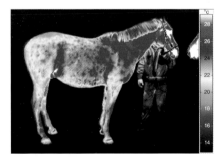

Fig. 1.7. Thermogram of the right lateral aspect of the horse. The warmest areas of the body are presented as white and red, yellow and green indicate cooler areas, and blue and black represent the coldest areas of the body.

or higher. Less noise, and therefore better accuracy, in a thermogram is provided by higher thermal sensitivity, which describes the smallest difference in temperature that a thermal imager can resolve between two points in the image. Many modern portable cameras have thermal sensitivities of less than 0.05°C: the smaller the value, the higher the sensitivity. When deciding on a thermographic camera, the basic functions of the camera need to be considered, as well as whether they will meet the requirements. All cameras can record single images, but some can also capture 'radiometric' video sequences, where each frame of the video can be analysed to extract temperature data. The ability to record standard visible-light photographs in the same imager may also be useful. Image capture to an on-board memory card is standard in most cameras; some can also stream data to mobile devices or computers via a USB cable or wirelessly. For anything more than the most basic evaluation of thermograms, thermographic image analysis software is required to adjust, analyse and report on the images recorded. Basic software may be included with the camera purchased, but more advanced analysis may be required and could entail further expenditure.

A thermal camera should undergo a regular programme of calibration for quality assurance to ensure that its output remains accurate. It is recommended that calibration be performed annually by the camera manufacturer. This calibration must be across a temperature range appropriate to equine thermography (e.g. 10–40°C), and should be traceable to the International Temperature Scale of 1990 (ITS-90). For research applications, requiring a high degree of accuracy and repeatability, it may be cost effective to purchase a 'blackbody' calibrator for in-house quality assurance of thermal images.

Technology moves rapidly, and recently phone applications have been developed that allow thermal images to be taken by the non-professional. Images taken with such new technologies must be viewed with caution, as the results are likely to be unreliable and erroneous for reasons that will become evident in the following chapters, in particular Chapter 2 (this volume).

1.6   Thermography as a Diagnostic Tool in Equine Medicine

The first thermographic cameras were produced in the early 1940s. In practice, they were initially used for military and industrial purposes (Rogalski, 2011), but from the middle of the 20th century, thermographic measurements began to play an important role in medical diagnostics (Ring, 2007). One of the first research studies investigated the use of thermography in diagnosing breast cancer (Lawson, 1956). From these early beginnings, thermographic techniques have developed for use in many other areas of medicine including inflammatory diseases, complex regional pain syndrome, Raynaud's phenomenon, burns and dermatology (Ring and Ammer, 2012).

The practical application of thermography in veterinary medicine began in the mid-1960s and early 1970s, with the first significant scientific publications appearing in the USA. The most significant authors at this time were R. Purohit, T. Turner, K. Bowman, L. Van Hoogmoed and J. Snyder, and their work provided the foundation for the use of thermography in veterinary medicine and the basis for further research applying this diagnostic tool to horses (Bowman *et al.*, 1983; Turner *et al.*, 1986; Van Hoogmoed *et al.*, 2000). One of the first sets of results of research on thermography application to veterinary medicine was presented by Smith (1964). On the basis of knowledge gained in human thermography, the author detected splints, bruised joints and bowed tendons. The paper presented by Delahanty and Georgi (1965) demonstrated the usefulness of thermography for detecting clinical cases of a squamous cell carcinoma, a slab fracture of the third metacarpal bone, a bone spavin and a deep cervical abscess.

Further studies investigated body temperature distribution characteristics of horses in specific ambient conditions. Such knowledge of body surface temperature distribution in the healthy horse is vitally important in the diagnosis of pathologies (Purohit and McCoy, 1980; Turner, 2001; Tunley and Henson, 2004).

1.7   Normal Body Surface Temperature Distribution of the Horse

The body surface (superficial) temperature distribution varies for each individual horse. The following factors (among others) influence body surface temperature values: anatomical structure, subcutaneous tissue, muscle tissue, hair coat and season of the year, as well as (in the case of sport horses) the training type and degree of animal adaptation to training load.

1.7.1   Anatomical structure

The body surface of a horse is both concave and convex, resulting in the emitted infrared radiation energy being unequal across the body surface (Cena and Clark, 1973). The concave parts of the body (e.g. the area around the base of the neck) or protected parts (e.g. the area behind the elbow joint) are less likely to be influenced by environmental factors. As a result, these areas have a higher body surface temperature. The surrounding more convex areas, such as the croup, are more exposed to the environment and so have a lower body surface temperature (Fig. 1.8).

1.7.2   Subcutaneous tissue

Thermal conduction from the surface vascular network arrangement and tissue metabolism has a major influence on body surface temperature (Draper and Boag, 1971a,b; Davy, 1977). Body areas with a higher tissue metabolism (e.g. shoulder, croup) have a higher temperature than areas with less tissue activity. The variation in surface temperature reflects changes in local perfusion, so skin, and hence the body surface temperature, overlying veins is normally warmer than that over arteries, because veins lie more superficially (e.g. jugular veins). The heat transferred by deeper-lying arteries and internal organs is significantly absorbed by subcutaneous tissues, which sometimes contain large amounts of

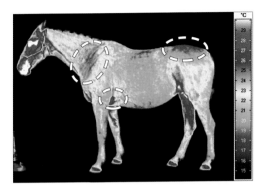

Fig. 1.8. Thermogram of the left lateral aspect of the horse. Concave body surface areas (such as the base of the neck area and the protected body surface at the elbow joint) are less exposed and so are less affected by environmental conditions and appear warmer compared with the croup area (dashed outlines).

accumulated fat. Hence, the distribution and quantity of subcutaneous tissues and fatty tissue layers affect body surface temperature distribution.

1.7.3 Muscle tissue

Muscle also influences body surface temperature. Body areas with muscle tissues, which have a rich blood supply (e.g. around the neck and upper forelimbs and hindlimbs), have a higher surface temperature compared with the less muscular areas (e.g. around the forearm and gaskin) and areas with no muscle (e.g. the distal forelimbs: from the carpal joint to the hoof (Fig. 1.9)).

1.7.4 Hair coat

Body surface temperature distribution also depends on hair coat. A thick coat strongly absorbs infrared radiation emitted from the skin surface (Cena and Monteith, 1975). Additionally, air is trapped in the hair coat, which, as a very poor heat conductor, creates an effective insulation against excessive heat loss. Therefore, the thickness, density, length and layout of the hair coat have a significant impact on temperature distribution (Cena and Clark, 1973; Clark and Cena, 1977). Body areas with thinner, less dense or shorter hair coats (e.g. the area around the head and flank) have a higher body surface temperature compared with areas with thicker, denser or longer hair coats (e.g. the area around the croup and pasterns; Fig. 1.9). One of the goals of clipping sport horses during the autumn and winter season is to facilitate thermoregulation by removing their thick winter hair coat. This treatment affects the body surface temperature, with the temperature in the clipped areas being higher compared with non-clipped areas (Fig. 1.10) (Turner et al., 1983).

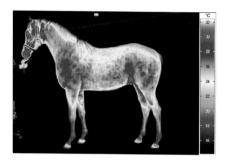

Fig. 1.9. Thermogram of the left lateral aspect of the horse. The warmest areas are the muscular areas at the neck and upper forelimbs and hindlimbs, whereas the coolest areas are those devoid of muscles – the distal limbs below the carpal joint. The hair coat also affects the body surface temperature. Areas of longer hair coat at the upper neck, spine, croup and pasterns are cooler than those with less hair coat.

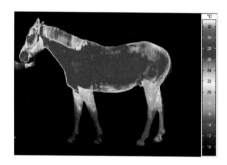

Fig. 1.10. Thermogram of the left lateral aspect of the horse. Clipped areas such as the neck, shoulder, chest and croup are warmer as a result of having less coat cover.

1.7.5   Season of the year

As might be expected, the body surface temperature distribution changes between summer and winter in relation to the length of the hair coat. In addition, during the summer season, 'warm spots' are visible on the thermogram, corresponding to areas of concentrated superficial blood vessels acting to increase heat exchange between the body and the environment, thus aiding cooling (Fig. 1.11). During the winter season, when the animal remains in an environment with low ambient temperatures, the hair coat becomes longer and thicker and vasoconstriction reduces blood flow in superficial blood vessels. As a result, the difference between the body surface temperature and the ambient temperature decreases and heat loss decreases accordingly (Fig. 1.12).

The absolute body surface temperature distribution of a horse is a highly individual trait, and is influenced by many environmental factors. It has been

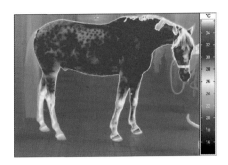

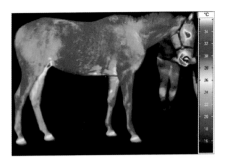

Fig. 1.11. Thermogram of the right lateral aspect of the horse. Influence of an elevated ambient temperature (20°C) on horse body surface temperature.

Fig. 1.12. Thermogram of the right lateral aspect of the horse. Influence of a reduced ambient temperature (10°C) on body surface temperature.

reported that body surface temperature across an individual horse can range from 19 up to 32°C. The highest body surface temperatures (27–32°C) have been reported to be on the head, neck, shoulder, upper arm, forearm and flank, and the lowest temperatures (24–26°C) on the distal limbs (Flores, 1978). However, Jodkowska and Dudek (2000) reported slightly different temperature ranges, with the range of highest temperatures (25–28°C) in the area of the head, middle part of the neck, chest and flanks, and the lowest temperatures (19–23°C) in the distal limbs. These differences in temperature ranges between studies highlight the effect and importance of different ambient temperatures.

2 Fundamentals of Thermographic Examination

2.1 Procedures for Thermographic Examination, Including the Impact of Environmental Conditions

Both internal and external factors have a significant effect on body surface temperature. The proper use of thermography to evaluate body surface thermal patterns therefore requires a controlled environment, and the physiological state of the horse must be considered in order to reduce variability and eliminate errors of interpretation (Head and Dyson, 2001; Purohit, 2009).

2.1.1 Preparing a room for thermographic examination

The thermographic examination should be performed indoors, in a stable ambient temperature on an appropriately prepared horse. It is important to take measurements within a specific ambient temperature range, as this will have a significant influence on the body surface temperature distribution (Purohit and McCoy, 1980; Palmer, 1983; Tunley and Henson, 2004). Extreme variations in environmental temperature may cause the body surface to show asymmetry in temperature distribution. The optimal ambient temperature of the examination room is approximately 20°C (Turner, 1991). Ambient temperatures above 25°C make it difficult to obtain a gradient (difference) between body surface temperature and the ambient temperature, and so local inflammation may be masked. Temperatures of 18–20°C may cause an increased but unevenly distributed blood flow arising from vasodilation in the distal forelimbs. If the ambient temperature is too low (below 15°C), vasoconstriction results in a decreased blood supply (Mogg and Pollitt, 1992). Temperatures below 12°C result in a general decrease in blood circulation, causing a reduction in body surface temperature. This is particularly seen in the distal limbs (Fig. 2.1) (Palmer, 1981, 1983).

© M. Soroko and M.C.G. Davies Morel 2016. *Equine Thermography in Practice*
(M. Soroko and M.C.G. Davies Morel)

Despite the ideal of 20°C, in practice thermographic examinations can be performed at a stable ambient temperature within a range of 12–25°C. The ambient temperature inside and outside the examination room should always be recorded.

Artefacts such as heat sources from sunlight, lamps and heaters should be eliminated (Palmer, 1981; Turner, 1991). Air draughts should also be avoided, as even barely noticeable air movements are able to decrease the body surface temperature, particularly of the limbs (Westermann *et al.*, 2013). Examples of artefacts affecting the body surface temperature distribution are presented in Figs 2.2–2.4.

The presence of high levels of dust particles in the air can interfere with infrared radiation. The dust reduces the quantity and quality of energy in the electromagnetic waves detected by the thermographic camera. Therefore, measurements should be taken in a well-ventilated room.

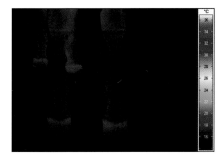

Fig. 2.1. Thermogram of the distal right and left forelimbs from the dorsal aspect. A low ambient temperature (10°C) decreases the body surface temperature in the distal part of both forelimbs.

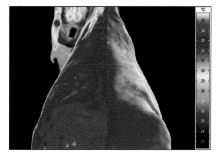

Fig. 2.2. Thermogram of the back and croup from the dorsal aspect. Sunlight has increased the body surface temperature in the area of the left side of the back and croup.

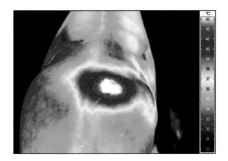

Fig. 2.3. Thermogram of the croup from the dorsal aspect. Sunlight has increased the body surface temperature in the area of the right side of the croup.

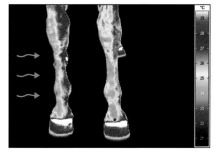

Fig. 2.4. Thermogram of the distal right and left forelimbs from the dorsal aspect. Air flow (in the direction indicated) from the right side of the horse has caused artefacts on the lateral and medial sides of the distal forelimbs.

Indoor thermography measurement standards have been established in equine veterinary practice. To enhance the diagnostic value of thermography, the following protocol should be adopted regarding the room used for imaging:

- The room temperature should be stabilized and maintained between 12 and 25°C (optimum around 20°C).
- The room should be draught free.
- The windows should be covered and the doors closed.

If there is no room that meets these requirements, thermographic examination can be performed in a wide, shaded stable corridor with a clean and even floor, although this is not ideal. Outdoor thermographic examination is not recommended because of the direct impact of the external environment, which will result in unreliable thermograms (Purohit, 2009; American Academy of Thermology, 2013).

2.1.2   Preparing a horse for thermographic examination

Thermographic examination of the horse should be performed at rest and before training, to avoid changes in body heat balance and blood circulation due to working muscles. However, in specific cases, thermographic examinations after exercise are also performed. It is recommended that the horse be acclimatized for 20 min prior to imaging in the room where thermography will take place. A longer period of equilibration may be required in cases where the animal is transported from an extremely cold or hot environment. According to Tunley and Henson (2004), the thermographic pattern does not change significantly during acclimatization, but the time taken for stabilization of the absolute temperature of the body surface is between 39 and 60 min. The major factor affecting this equilibration time is the temperature difference between the original environment and that in which the images are to be obtained. Therefore, a longer stabilization period of 1 h is suggested after exposure to a very different ambient temperature to that in which the image is to be taken (Palmer, 1983). It should also be noted that a horse with a long coat will require a longer acclimatization time than a clipped horse or one with a short coat.

Standards for indoor thermography measurement have been established in equine veterinary practice. To enhance the diagnostic value of thermography, the following protocols should be adopted regarding the preparation of the horse:

- Allow adequate acclimatization time prior to imaging; in spring and summer this is approximately 20 min, while in autumn and winter it is 1 h.
- The horse should be examined at rest (which should be after at least 3 h of rest and before training) (Turner et al., 2001). Ideally this should be in the morning, after the horse has rested in the stable.
- The horse must have a clean, dry hair coat and should be groomed at least 1 h before the examination.

Variables in winter hair coats can confuse interpretation (von Schweinitz, 1999). It has been found that clipping does not cause any change in the thermal distribution but does result in an increase in overall body surface temperature. Therefore, clipping is not required to produce reliable thermographic images, but it is necessary that the hair coat be short and of uniform length and that it lies flat against the skin to permit thermal conduction (Turner *et al.*, 1983). A horse should be dry when presented for imaging, as a wet or damp hair coat decreases the body surface temperature. The feet should also be clean, the hooves picked out and the body, limbs and feet brushed to remove external contamination, without any ointments applied. Systemic or topical medications should not be applied prior to imaging, and any residues should be washed off the previous day (Turner, 1991). This also applies to direct covers and dressings, such as boots or bandages, which, when attached to the distal limbs, can result in elevated body surface temperatures for prolonged periods of time (Fig. 2.5).

Rugs, blankets and other coverings should be removed at least 30 min before the examination (Palmer, 1981). Elastic cloths made of Lycra® and fitted under rugs should be taken off a day before the examination, because they adhere strongly to the horse's body (Fig. 2.6) and affect the body surface temperature.

The mane should be platted before the examination; otherwise, it will absorb the infrared radiation from the covered part of the neck (Fig. 2.7). The tail should also be platted and protected.

Local changes to the hair coat due to damage or tearing result in an increased body surface temperature compared with the surrounding area (Figs 2.8 and 2.9). In some cases, freeze branding affects the body surface temperature due to skin nerve damage (Fig. 2.10). Scars after injury or veterinary treatment also influence the body surface temperature.

The horse should not receive any physical therapy in the 24-h period prior to the thermographic examination. Treatments such as a warm (40°C) or cold (4°C) gel wrap to the distal limb can have a significant effect. Such cold therapy is reported to result in temperature differences of 2.5°C between treated and untreated limbs 2 h after treatment (Eddy *et al.*, 2001). A heated wrap resulted in a temperature difference between the limbs that actually increased with time after

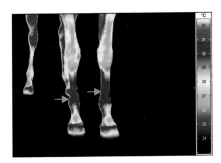

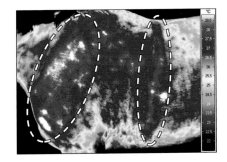

Fig. 2.5. Thermogram of the distal part of the right and left forelimbs from the dorsal aspect. An increased body surface temperature of the right and left third metacarpal bones (green arrows) is evident following removal of bandages from both forelimbs 2 h earlier.

Fig. 2.6. Thermogram of the left side of the shoulder and chest from the lateral aspect. An increased body surface temperature of the left aspect of the shoulder and chest in the area where clinging elastic cloths (fitted under the rug) were applied is indicated (dashed outlines).

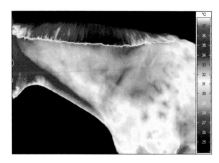

Fig. 2.7. Thermogram of the left side of neck from the lateral aspect. The mane absorbs infrared radiation emissions from the neck area, which appears cooler as a result.

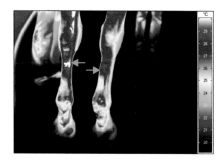

Fig. 2.8. Thermogram of the distal part of the right and left forelimbs from the palmar aspect. A local increased body surface temperature is evident in the area of the right and left third metacarpal bone (blue arrows), because of hair coat damage caused by wearing boots.

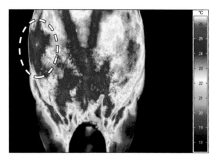

Fig. 2.9. Thermogram of the chest from the dorsal aspect. A local increased body surface temperature is evident in the area of the right shoulder joint (dashed outline) due to hair coat damage caused by wearing a rug.

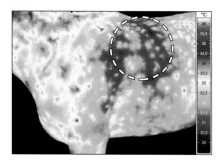

Fig. 2.10. Thermogram of the left shoulder and chest from the lateral aspect, illustrating the effect of branding on reducing the body surface temperature (dashed outline).

removal. Thirty minutes after removal of the wrap, the temperature difference was 2.8°C, which increased to 3.7°C after 75 min. It has also been reported that therapeutic ultrasound applied to the flexor tendon region for 10 min significantly increases the temperature of the treated limb for more than 1 h. However, biomagnetic therapy to flexor tendons for 24 h is reported to have no effect on body surface temperature. Additionally, acupuncture treatment should be avoided for at least 1 week before thermographic examination.

If medical treatment of a horse is planned, the thermographic examination should be performed beforehand, as sedatives and anti-inflammatory or anaesthetic agents have an effect on superficial blood circulation, changing the body surface temperature. Clipping the body in preparation for ultrasound examination will also distort the results (Fig. 2.11). Similarly nerve blocking, neurectomy, skin lesions such as scars or blisters, or surgically

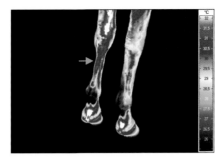

Fig. 2.11. Thermogram of the distal right and left forelimbs from the palmar aspect. A local increased body surface temperature in the area of the left third metacarpal bone (blue arrow) is evident due to localized clipping prior to ultrasound.

altered areas also affect the body surface temperature (Purohit, 2008). Artefacts can be produced by any material on the body surface such as dirt, thick coat, scars and bands (Palmer, 1981).

Additional digital photographs may be taken at the same time to support the thermographic examination records.

2.1.3   Interview with the horse owner

Asking the horse owner to complete a questionnaire to give additional information may be helpful in informing which thermographic images should be taken, the measurements to be made and ultimately their interpretation. The first part of the questionnaire should include basic information about the horse: age, gender, breed, type of performance and current training programme, plus any training and saddle-fit problems. The questionnaire should also provide information on hoof function, current health problems and any previous injuries of the musculoskeletal system. A medical history is also required, including the results of other veterinary examinations such as radiography, ultrasonography and palpation. This is crucial because many musculoskeletal injuries can be detected by thermography not only in the acute or chronic phase but also the subclinical stage of inflammation. The second part of the questionnaire should describe the environmental conditions in the room during the thermographic examination. The third part of the questionnaire should contain information about the preparation of the horse for the examination: time to acclimatize, characterization of the hair coat and information on the presence of rugs, bandages, etc. before examination. A sample equine thermographic examination questionnaire is provided in Appendix 1.

2.2   Taking Images of the Horse

Adhering to a strict, repeatable protocol is important in order to ensure accurate interpretation of the images.

2.2.1 Thermographic protocol

The thermographic examination of the horse is normally undertaken with the horse at rest in order to increase the reliability of the body surface temperature distribution. In some cases, it is worth repeating the thermographic examination after exercise (lunging or riding), especially if there are difficulties in identifying the site of injury. If this is the case, a body surface temperature change may be seen after the training load. For example, Vaden *et al.* (1980) reported that abnormal thermograms of tarsal joint osteoarthritis were more distinct after exercise. An increased blood supply to the affected digit resulted in dilation of the capillaries and larger blood vessels and a higher body surface temperature. Similarly, a lack of proper muscle balance during training may indicate a problem, which will be clearly visible immediately after exercise. A single image will often suffice, but commonly images of symmetrical parts of the body, e.g. lateral images of the left and right sides of the horse, are required to allow comparisons to be made.

The essence of reliable thermographic measurements is keeping the same measurement conditions. This particularly applies to the following:

*   Reproducible horse positioning.
*   A consistent distance between the camera and the horse; keeping the same distance is especially important for symmetrical parts of the body taken in two separate thermographic images.
*   Proper focusing of each thermographic image.

2.2.2 Correct positioning of the horse and camera

The thermographic images can be recorded from a camera mounted on a tripod, or from a 'handheld' device, keeping the camera lens perpendicular to the centre of the examined body area. Thermograms should be captured at an appropriate distance (Table 2.1), always keeping the distance between the examined animal and the camera constant.

To help maintain a consistent distance between the camera and the horse, the floor can be marked. An equal imaging distance for symmetrical parts of the body taken in two separate images is crucial for correct comparison of the left and right sides. A change in imaging distance (even by half a metre) for symmetrical parts of the body can contribute to inconsistent temperature readings

Table 2.1. Recommended distance between horse and camera for specific body areas of a horse.

Body area	Distance (m)
Distal limbs	1–1.5
Back and croup of the horse from the dorsal aspect	1.5–2
Head, neck, shoulder, chest and croup area from the lateral aspect	2
Lateral aspect of the horse body	7

due to the limitations of camera optics and detectors. Figures 2.12 and 2.13 illustrate the croup area of a horse taken from different distances. When the camera is positioned at 2 m away from the horse, the croup area appears to have a higher body surface temperature (Fig. 2.12) than when the camera is positioned 3 m away (Fig. 2.13).

Symmetrical parts of the body in one thermographic image (e.g. both limbs) should be positioned next to each other; the horse should stand straight without lateral and medial rotation, and the limbs should be evenly loaded. Figures 2.14 and 2.15 illustrate incorrect limb positioning (unevenly loaded).

Symmetrical body parts presented in two separate thermographic images (e.g. the left and right sides of the neck) should have the same positioning in relation to the camera. Figure 2.16 illustrates incorrect positioning of the neck in relation to the camera, in which the right side of the neck is bent away from the camera. Figure 2.17 presents the correct neck position in relation to the camera.

It is also important to position the part of the body being examined in the centre of the frame and to ensure that the focusing is correct, as this cannot be corrected by the analysis software after imaging. In contrast, the colour palette

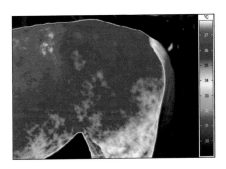

Fig. 2.12. Thermogram of the left side of the croup from the lateral aspect, taken from a distance of 2 m from the horse.

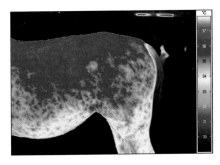

Fig. 2.13. Thermogram of the left side of the croup from the lateral aspect, taken from a distance of 3 m from the horse.

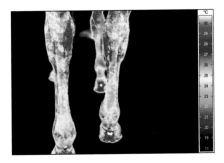

Fig. 2.14. Thermogram of the distal part of the right and left hindlimbs from the plantar aspect. The limbs are not evenly loaded.

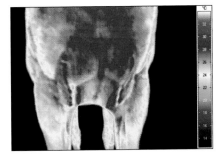

Fig. 2.15. Thermogram of the chest from the dorsal aspect. The forelimbs not evenly loaded so the right limb is forward compared with the left. This results in asymmetry, with the left chest area appearing smaller than the right chest area.

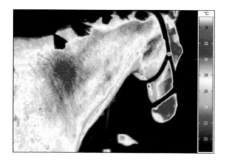
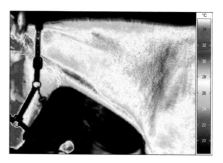

Fig. 2.16. Thermogram of the right side of the neck from the lateral aspect, illustrating an incorrect neck position in relation to the camera (the neck is turned to the left side).

Fig. 2.17. Thermogram of the left side of the neck from lateral aspect, illustrating the correct neck position in relation to the camera.

and range of temperatures included in each thermogram can usually be modified using the computer software. The temperature range should be adjusted to include the full range of temperatures encountered across the horse, and should be applied to each image consistently, particularly when comparing symmetrical parts of the body. Automatic settings for the temperature range, applied by the camera for each image, should be avoided as they afford no user control of the temperature scale.

2.2.3   Sample thermographic images

Sample thermographic images recorded from a healthy horse at rest in stabilized environmental conditions are presented in the following sections. These thermograms show the whole lateral aspect of the horse as well as selected areas: the distal forelimbs and hindlimbs, and the shoulder, croup, chest, neck and head areas.

When undertaking thermographic examination, it is very important to take images of the whole horse utilizing the entire protocol as described below, as a problem appearing in one part of the body may be caused by dysfunctions of the musculoskeletal system (muscles, tendons, ligaments and bones) in other areas.

The basic thermographic images of the examined horse as described below may be supplemented by additional images. Depending on the problem, it may also be appropriate to take images before and after exercise and/or close-up images of regions of interest from different aspects. Repeated scans of suspected areas over time may also be useful and yield more reliable information.

Interpretation of the thermographic images using computer software is discussed in Chapter 3 (this volume).

2.2.3.1   Lateral aspect of the horse
Figures 2.18 and 2.19 show both lateral aspects of the whole horse and are basic thermograms presenting the overall body surface temperature distribution. The horse in this image is standing with one limb in front of the other so that

the lateral and medial aspects of the distal limbs are visible from both sides. The distance between the horse and the camera should be about 7 m (Table 2.1).

2.2.3.2 Distal forelimbs

Basic imaging of the distal forelimbs should be focused on the limb area between the carpal joint and the hoof. A single thermographic image should include both limbs from the dorsal aspect (Fig. 2.20), followed by separate thermographic images of:

- the right forelimb from the lateral aspect and the left forelimb from the medial aspect (Fig. 2.21);
- the left forelimb from the lateral aspect and the right forelimb from the medial aspect (Fig. 2.22); and
- the right and left forelimb from the palmar aspect imaged from both the right (Fig. 2.23) and the left (Fig. 2.24) side of the horse.

Measurement of the distal parts of the forelimbs should be performed from a consistent distance of approximately 1–1.5 m (Table 2.1).

2.2.3.3 Distal hindlimbs

Basic imaging of the distal hindlimbs should be focused on the limb area between the tarsal joint and the hoof. A single thermographic image should

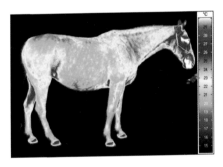

Fig. 2.18. Thermogram of the right lateral aspect of the horse.

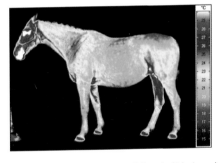

Fig. 2.19. Thermogram of the left lateral aspect of the horse.

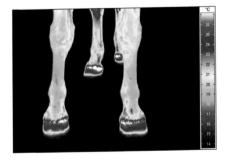

Fig. 2.20. Thermogram of the distal right and left forelimbs from the dorsal aspect.

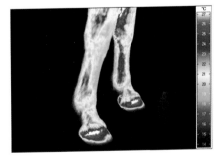

Fig. 2.21. Thermogram of the distal right and left forelimbs from the lateral and medial aspects, respectively (from the right side of the horse).

include both limbs from the plantar aspect (Fig. 2.25), followed by separate thermographic images of:

- the right hindlimb from the dorsal aspect (Fig. 2.26);
- the left hindlimb from the dorsal aspect (Fig. 2.27);

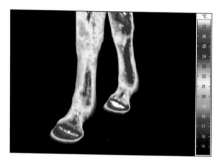

Fig. 2.22. Thermogram of the distal left and right forelimbs from the lateral and medial aspects, respectively (from the left side of the horse).

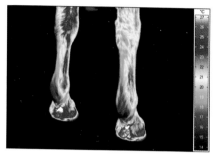

Fig. 2.23. Thermogram of the distal right and left forelimbs from the palmar aspect (from the right side of the horse).

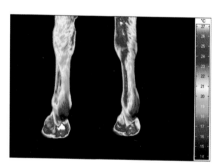

Fig. 2.24. Thermogram of the distal left and right forelimbs from the palmar aspect (from the left side of the horse).

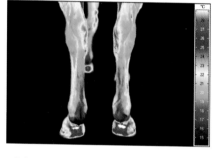

Fig. 2.25. Thermogram of the distal right and left hindlimbs from the plantar aspect.

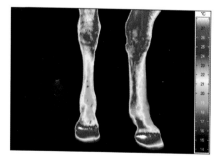

Fig. 2.26. Thermogram of the distal right hindlimb from the dorsal aspect.

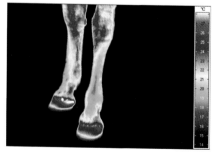

Fig. 2.27. Thermogram of the distal left hindlimb from the dorsal aspect.

- the right hindlimb from the lateral aspect and the left hindlimb from the medial aspect (Fig. 2.28); and
- the left hindlimb from the lateral aspect and the right hindlimb from the medial aspect (Fig. 2.29).

Measurement of the distal hindlimb should be performed from a consistent distance of approximately 1–1.5 m (Table 2.1).

2.2.3.4 Shoulder area
Basic imaging of the upper part of the forelimbs is focused on the shoulder area (Figs 2.30 and 2.31). A thermogram of the shoulder area from the lateral aspect should include the following body areas: withers, base of the neck, shoulder and elbow joints. The distance between the camera and the shoulder area should be around 2 m and consistent on both sides (Table 2.1).

2.2.3.5 Croup area
Basic imaging of the upper part of the hindlimbs is focused on the croup area. A thermogram of the croup area from the lateral aspect should include the following body areas: flank, sacral and coccygeal vertebrae, and stifle joint (Figs 2.32 and 2.33). A thermogram of this body area from the dorsal aspect

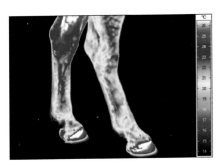

Fig. 2.28. Thermogram of the distal right and left hindlimbs from the lateral and medial aspects, respectively (from the right side of the horse).

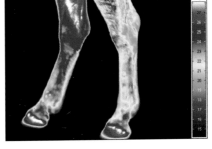

Fig. 2.29. Thermogram of the distal left and right hindlimbs from the lateral and medial aspects, respectively (from the left side of the horse).

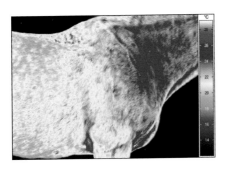

Fig. 2.30. Thermogram of the right side of the shoulder from the lateral aspect.

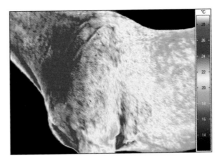

Fig. 2.31. Thermogram of the left side of the shoulder from the lateral aspect.

should include the following body areas: sacroiliac joints, sacral vertebrae, pelvis (including tuber coxae) and dock (Fig. 2.34). The croup area from the caudal aspect should include the body area between the dock and stifle joint (Fig. 2.35). The distance between the camera and the lateral aspect of the croup area should be around 2 m and consistent on both sides. For the caudal aspect, the imaging distance should be also 2 m, and for the dorsal aspect, it should be around 1.5–2 m (Table 2.1).

2.2.3.6 Chest area

Basic imaging of the chest area is shown in Figs 2.36 and 2.37. A thermogram of the chest area from the lateral aspect should include the following body areas: back (thoracic and lumbar vertebrae), barrel including flank and elbow joint area. The distance between the camera and the chest area should be around 2 m and consistent on both sides (Table 2.1).

2.2.3.7 Neck area

Basic imaging for the neck area is shown in Figs 2.38 and 2.39. A thermogram of neck area from the lateral aspect should include the area between the base of the neck and the poll. The distance between the camera and the neck area should be around 2 m and consistent on both sides (Table 2.1).

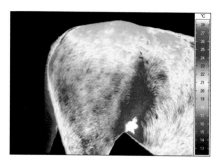

Fig. 2.32. Thermogram of the right side of the croup from the lateral aspect.

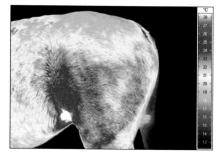

Fig. 2.33. Thermogram of the left side of the croup from the lateral aspect.

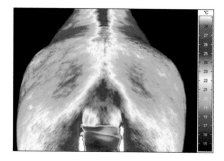

Fig. 2.34. Thermogram of the croup from the dorsal aspect.

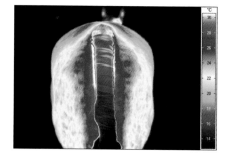

Fig. 2.35. Thermogram of the croup from the caudal aspect.

2.2.3.8 Head area

Basic imaging of the head area is shown in Figs 2.40 and 2.41. A thermogram of the head area should include the whole lateral aspect of the head. The distance between the camera and the head area should be around 2 m and consistent on both sides (Table 2.1).

2.2.3.9 Back area

Basic imaging of the back is shown in Fig. 2.42. A thermogram of the back from the dorsal aspect should include the thoracic and lumbar vertebrae. The images

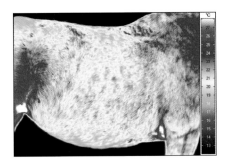

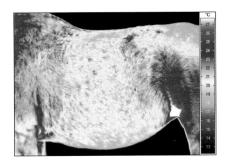

Fig. 2.36. Thermogram of the right side of the chest from the lateral aspect.

Fig. 2.37. Thermogram of the left side of the chest from the lateral aspect.

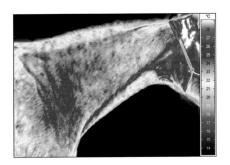

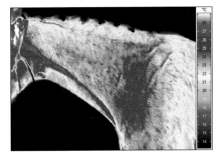

Fig. 2.38. Thermogram of the right side of the neck from the lateral aspect.

Fig. 2.39. Thermogram of the left side of the neck from the lateral aspect.

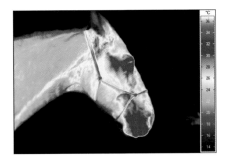

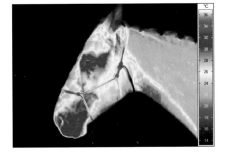

Fig. 2.40. Thermogram of the right side of the head from the lateral aspect.

Fig. 2.41. Thermogram of the left side of the head from the lateral aspect.

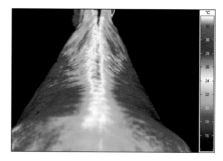

Fig. 2.42. Thermogram of the back from the dorsal aspect.

in this area are taken from a height of approximately 3 m off of the ground using a ladder placed 1.5 m behind the horse.

2.3 Most Frequently Made Errors in Thermographic Imaging

The most frequent errors in thermographic imaging include the following:

- Incorrect preparation of the examination room to minimize artefacts, such as sunlight, draughts, etc.
- Taking thermographic images on an uneven or wet floor.
- Only removing rugs or bandages just before the examination.
- Inadequate acclimatization time prior to the imaging.
- Touching the horse during or just before measurements.
- Changing the environmental conditions during imaging.
- Stopping the measurement and beginning again after a delay.
- Incorrect positioning of the horse in relation to the camera.
- Failure to maintain a consistent distance between the camera and the horse.
- Failure to employ a consistent or appropriate temperature scale on the thermogram.
- Uneven positioning of symmetrical limbs in one thermographic image.
- Uneven loading of the limbs by the horse.
- Imaging with incorrect focusing.
- The body part for examination not being positioned in the centre of the frame.
- An insufficient number of images.
- No detailed interview on the current and previous health of the horse, or on the current training programme.

3

Interpretation of Thermographic Images and the Normal Superficial Temperature Distribution of the Horse

3.1 Thermography Analysis for Veterinary or Prophylactic Purposes

Thermographic image analysis is carried out by specialized computer software invariably purchased with the thermographic camera. The program also enables modifications to be made to the thermogram, including changes to the colour palette and temperature range. The software can also be used to calculate the temperature of selected body areas on each thermogram, and to add comments. The type of image analysis depends on the manner and goal of the thermographic examination.

3.2 Analysis of Symmetry and Repeatability of Body Surface Temperature Distribution in Contralateral Body Areas of the Horse

As the horse is bilaterally symmetrical, there is normally a high degree of right and left symmetry of temperature distribution on the horse. A number of studies have reported repeatable body surface temperature distribution on different horses (Purohit and McCoy, 1980; Palmer, 1981). This allows the creation of a map of the normal temperature distribution of the symmetrical parts of the body of a horse at rest under controlled environmental conditions against which abnormalities can be assessed. The symmetry of temperature distribution and the repeatability of temperature maps are, however, very strongly influenced by the anatomy, breed and training of a horse. Thermogram analysis based only on repeatable temperature maps may therefore be misleading due to changing environmental conditions, as well as variations such as hair coat. A good example is the different body surface temperature distribution in summer and

© M. Soroko and M.C.G. Davies Morel 2016. *Equine Thermography in Practice*
(M. Soroko and M.C.G. Davies Morel)

winter (see Figs 1.11 and 1.12, Chapter 1, this volume). Therefore, analysis of symmetrical body surface temperature distribution in a single image, or using two images, one of each side of the horse taken under identical conditions at the same time, is the main requirement for thermographic image interpretation.

3.2.1 Determination of body surface temperature differences between symmetrical body areas or regions of interest (ROIs)

A difference in symmetry of body surface temperature between ROIs on the opposite sides of the horse is a successful way of identifying abnormalities. This difference may be obvious to the naked eye if all thermograms are presented with the same temperature scale so that temperature differences can be quantified. Additionally, specific regions of the horse that are of particular interest can be identified by circles, lines or specifically drawn areas, and programmed into the software to appear on the thermograms as ROIs. Within each ROI, the analysis software can determine the average temperature value. Symmetrical ROIs, such as in the case of left and right distal limbs, can then easily be compared (Fig. 3.1). This is a thermographic examination methodology commonly used in commercial practice and in research (Tunley and Henson, 2004; Soroko et al., 2013).

Average temperature differences of greater than 1°C between symmetrical ROIs on the distal limb are reported to indicate inflammation (Turner, 1991; Soroko et al., 2013). However, the International Equestrian Federation (FEI) regulations have determined a threshold difference for inflammation of 2°C (International Equestrian Federation, 2015).

It has also been reported that temperature differences of 1.25°C between distal limbs can indicate subclinical inflammation of the superficial digital flexor tendon and bucked shins in racehorses (Soroko et al., 2013). A further study (Turner, 1991) suggested that the early stages of bucked shins could be diagnosed when local temperatures over the dorsal third metacarpal bone

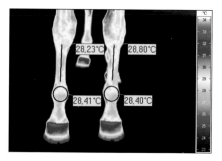

Fig. 3.1. Thermogram of the distal right and left forelimbs from the dorsal aspect, with the average temperature of the symmetrical linear bars and circular ROIs shown, allowing quantified comparisons to be made.

were 1–2°C higher compared with the surrounding distal limb areas. In the early phase of laminitis, the coronary band may show a significantly increased surface temperature (1–2°C) compared with the distal hoof and sole (Turner, 1991). Laminitis may be further indicated when the temperature of the hoof matches the elevated temperature of the coronary band (Turner, 2003). Care must be taken, however, as asymmetry in body surface temperature of the distal limbs may, under certain circumstances, be normal and not indicative of pathology. This was indicated in a study by Palmer (1983), where skin surface temperatures were taken at three different ambient temperatures (5, 15 and 25°C). In 88% of cases, the pairs of temperatures taken from symmetrical limb regions differed by 1°C or less. However, a few symmetrical readings differed by up to 5.5°C in the absence of any clinical signs of inflammation or lameness. While such asymmetry may be explained in terms of normal biological responses, the possibility of subclinical inflammation at these sites could not be excluded. Therefore, an understanding of normal temperature variations is crucial for interpretation of thermograms. In the case of the back, inflammation is indicated by an average ROI temperature difference of over 3°C between the spine and the back muscles. For other body areas containing muscle tissue, a similar 3°C difference in average temperature values between symmetrical ROIs is considered to be indicative of inflammation (Table 3.1).

This use of thermography to assess symmetry of surface body temperatures between symmetrical body areas is the prime means by which abnormalities in individual horses are diagnosed.

3.2.2 Determination of body surface temperature along linear ROIs or at specific points on the body surface

Body surface temperature along a linear ROI or at a point ROI can also be identified. These measurements are used to determine the presence of temperature differences between individual body areas on the same side of the horse, rather than comparison of symmetrical areas.

Table 3.1. Minimum differences in average temperature between symmetrical ROIs indicative of inflammation in a horse at rest.

Body area	Differences in average temperature between symmetrical body areas that are indicative of inflammation, according to Turner (1991), Tunley and Henson (2004) and Soroko et al. (2013)	Differences in average temperature between symmetrical body areas that are indicative of inflammation according to the FEI
Distal limbs	1°C	2°C
Spine (including back area)	3°C	–
Rest of the body	3°C	–

Linear body surface temperature measurements indicate that the warmest average surface temperature measurements along a line are: from the chest to the withers area, from the shoulder joint to the withers area, from the shoulder joint to the elbow joint, from the shoulder joint to the croup area and from the croup to the flank area. Conversely, the lowest temperatures are evident along a line down the distal hindlimbs and forelimbs (Fig. 3.2.; Jodkowska and Dudek, 2000).

Point body surface temperature measurements have indicated that the highest temperature is at the head area (eyes, nostrils and muzzle), neck, barrel and in the upper parts of the limbs: above the carpal joint in the forelimb and above the tarsal joint in the hindlimb (Fig. 3.3). The lowest temperatures are measured in the distal limbs (Jodkowska and Dudek, 2000). The difference in temperature between the warmest and coldest body surface areas is dependent on environmental conditions during the thermographic examination, primarily the ambient temperature. This type of measurement can be helpful to determine the change of temperature range between the individual points in relation to the ambient temperature.

Linear and point body surface temperature measurements are used in scientific research along with accompanying statistical analysis, and as such they need to be performed on a large group of horses. They do not apply to individual cases, where the goal of thermographic examination is diagnosis, treatment or prevention. In individual cases it is important to base the thermographic analysis on symmetry and repeatability of the body surface temperature distribution of the horse at rest.

3.2.3 Interpretation of thermograms

For the correct interpretation of thermograms, it is essential to consider the anatomy of the horse, particularly the muscle and bone structure, along with the neurological and blood circulation systems. Variability in the symmetry of temperature distribution may be due not only to local blood supply changes,

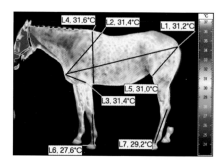

Fig. 3.2. Thermogram of the left lateral aspect of the horse, with the average temperature along the linear ROIs shown.

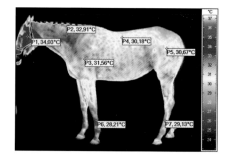

Fig. 3.3. Thermogram of the left lateral aspect of the horse, with point body temperature measurements shown.

indicative of inflammation, but also to the influence of the external environment, physical exercise, etc. Therefore, understanding normal variation in body surface temperature distribution is crucial for interpretation of thermograms.

The normal ranges of temperature differences between symmetrical parts of the body for the healthy horse are presented in Table 3.2. These temperature differences were determined on healthy horses at rest at an ambient environmental temperature of around 20°C. These values were determined on the basis of the author's observations of a group of 30 horses and are in agreement with other published results (Purohit and McCoy, 1980; Verschooten *et al.*, 1997; Turner, 2003; Tunley and Henson, 2004). These differences are subject to change if the images are taken in ambient temperatures below 12°C or above 25°C.

Body surface temperature distribution of a horse is characterized by the variability of individual features and is influenced by changing environmental

Table 3.2. Permissible temperature differences between symmetrical structures in specified parts of the body for a healthy horse.

Body area	Structure in specified part of the body	Permissible temperature difference
Distal parts of limbs	Coronary band	1–2°C higher compared with the rest of the hoof
	Hoof bar	2°C higher compared with the rest of hoof sole structures
	Area between the heel bulbs	5°C higher compared with the surrounding area
Back	Spine	Maximum of 3°C higher compared with the surrounding area
Shoulder	Shoulder joint	1.5°C lower compared with the surrounding area
	Elbow joint	1.5°C lower compared with the surrounding area
	Area behind elbow joint	1°C higher compared with the surrounding area
	Area in front of scapula	1°C higher compared with the surrounding area
Neck	Cervical vertebrae	1–1.5 lower compared with the surrounding area
	Jugular groove	2°C higher compared with the surrounding area
Head	Temporomandibular joint	3°C lower compared with the eye
Croup	Dorsal croup area	1°C lower compared with the surrounding area
	Stifle joint	1.5°C lower compared with the surrounding area
	Flank	2°C higher compared with the surrounding area

conditions. Hence, the determination of absolute normal surface body temperature distribution is not possible. Thermogram interpretation should therefore be based on body surface temperature distribution symmetry and on an understanding of the surface temperature map, indicating the expected difference in surface body temperature at each area. It must always take into consideration individual variation as well as the physiological condition of the examined horse.

The following sections detail the interpretation of thermograms for various parts of the body. In order to illustrate and clarify the correlation between body surface temperature distribution and the anatomy of the horse, the location of bones and joints is marked on the illustrative thermograms, and the major muscles are indicated on additional figures. In interpretation of the thermographic images of the distal limbs, their anatomy is considered in detail, including tendons, ligaments and blood vessels. All the following thermographic images were taken on a healthy horse at rest by the author and are in agreement with other published results (Purohit and McCoy, 1980; Turner, 2003; Tunley and Henson, 2004).

3.2.3.1   Distal forelimbs and hindlimbs

The most reproducible thermographic measurements can be achieved from the distal forelimbs and hindlimbs, because of the lack of thermogenic muscle tissue in the distal limb. Therefore, imaging is normally concentrated in that area. Several studies have presented surface temperature maps that have been correlated with the position of the individual structures of the limb (Purohit and McCoy, 1980; Vaden et al., 1980; Turner, 1991).

The distal forelimb from the carpal joint to the hoof and the hindlimb from the tarsal joint to the hoof are devoid of muscle. Movement is controlled via long tendons originating in muscles located in the upper or superior limb. These are the muscles located at the level of the radius (forelimbs) and the tibia (hindlimbs), which drive the motion of the distal limbs. The anatomy of these parts of the distal limbs means that the major structures (i.e. tendons, ligaments and blood vessels) can clearly be identified on the thermographic image. The tendons consist of dense fibrous connective tissue, predominantly composed of collagen fibres (which are the basic units responsible for the strength). Tendon tissue is characterized by a significant stretch strength and poor blood circulation. The main tendon at the palmar/plantar aspect of the third metacarpal/metatarsal bone is the superficial digital flexor tendon, and located beneath this is the deep digital flexor tendon. Both structures are responsible for flexion of the digit joints (Figs 3.4–3.7 and 3.9–3.10). At the dorsal aspect of the third metacarpal/metatarsal bone, the common digital extensor (forelimb; Fig. 3.4) and long digital extensor (hindlimb; Fig. 3.5) tendons are located. The main function of these tendons is extension of the digit joints (Figs 3.4, 3.5, 3.8 and 3.11). The distal limbs also consist of numerous ligaments connecting the bones, and supporting the joints. The suspensory ligament is located just behind the third metacarpal/metatarsal bone, under the deep digital flexor tendon (an example of this ligament is visible in Figs 3.4–3.6). The main function of this ligament is to support and stabilize the fetlock joint.

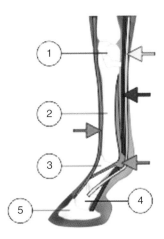

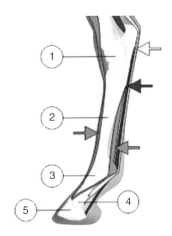

Fig. 3.4. Distal forelimb from the lateral aspect showing the carpus joint (1), third metacarpal bone (2), long pastern (3), short pastern (4), coffin bone (5), superficial digital flexor tendon (yellow arrow), deep digital flexor tendon (red arrow), common digital extensor tendon (green arrow) and suspensory ligament (blue arrow).

Fig. 3.5. Distal hindlimb from the lateral aspect showing the tarsus joint (1), third metatarsal bone (2), long pastern (3), short pastern (4), coffin bone (5), superficial digital flexor tendon (yellow arrow), deep digital flexor tendon (red arrow), long digital extensor tendon (green arrow) and suspensory ligament (blue arrow).

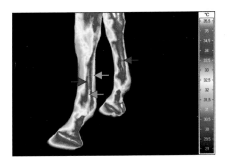

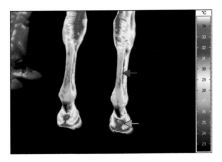

Fig. 3.6. Thermogram of the distal right and left forelimbs from the lateral and medial aspects, respectively. The palmar digital arteries of the right forelimb from the medial aspect and the palmar veins of the left forelimb from the lateral aspect (red arrows), suspensory ligament (blue arrow), superficial and deep digital flexor tendons (green arrow) are indicated.

Fig. 3.7. Thermogram of the distal right and left forelimbs from the palmar aspect with the superficial and deep digital flexor tendons (red arrow) and area between the heel bulbs (green arrow) indicated.

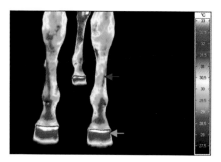

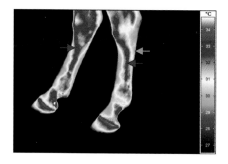

Fig. 3.8. Thermogram of the distal part of the right and left forelimbs from the dorsal aspect with the common digital extensor tendon (red arrow) and coronary band (green arrow) indicated.

Fig. 3.9. Thermogram of the distal right and left hindlimbs from the lateral and medial aspects respectively. The plantar digital artery of the right hindlimb from the medial aspect and plantar veins of the left hindlimb from the lateral aspect (red arrows) and superficial and deep digital flexor tendons (green arrow) indicated.

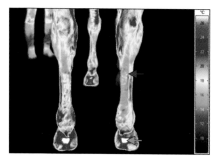

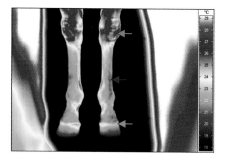

Fig. 3.10. Thermogram of the distal right and left hindlimbs from the plantar aspect with the superficial and deep digital flexor tendons (red arrow) and area between the heel bulbs (green arrow) indicated.

Fig. 3.11. Thermogram of the distal right and left hindlimbs from the dorsal aspect with the cooler long digital extensor tendon (green arrow) and coronary band (red arrow) and warmer tarsal joint (blue arrow) indicated.

The warmest areas of the forelimbs, including the metacarpal bones and the fetlock and pastern joints, are along the main blood vessels: the palmar and digital arteries, and also the palmar veins from the lateral and medial aspects (Fig. 3.6). Similarly, the warmest areas in the hindlimbs including the metatarsal bones, and the fetlock and pastern joints are along the plantar and digital arteries, and also the plantar veins from the lateral and medial aspects (Fig. 3.9) (Vaden *et al.*, 1980; Turner, 1991).

The areas of the metacarpal and metatarsal bones and the fetlock and pastern joints from the dorsal and palmar/plantar aspects appear cold on the thermographic image because they are located away from major blood vessels (Turner, 1991). The lower temperature of these areas is associated with the localization of the extensor and flexor tendons of the digit joints, which have a poor blood supply (Figs 3.7, 3.8, 3.10 and 3.11) (Turner *et al.*, 1996). The joints of the distal limb from the dorsal aspect are cooler than the surrounding structures with the exception of the tarsal joint, which is warmer on the dorsal aspect due to the superficial crossing of the cranial branch of the medial saphenous vein (Fig. 3.11) (Vaden *et al.*, 1980). The highest temperature in the distal parts of the limbs is in the coronary band, as it is situated close to the major arteriovenous plexus (Figs 3.8, 3.11 and 3.12; Kold and Chappell, 1998; Turner, 2001). The coronary band is warmer by 1–2°C compared with the hoof wall, which exhibits a gradually decreasing surface temperature towards the hoof sole (Fig. 3.12) (Verschooten *et al.*, 1997). The hoof sole from the solar aspect has a uniform temperature distribution across the sole, frog and heel bulb (Fig. 3.13). Only the hoof bars are characterized by a higher temperature – a maximum of 3°C warmer than the surrounding hoof sole. A raised temperature is also recorded in the area between the heel bulbs, which, due to the lack of hair, has a temperature 5°C higher than the surrounding body areas (Figs. 3.7 and 3.10).

Increased or decreased blood flow can be detected most reliably at the major blood vessels in the distal limbs from the lateral and medial aspects. In contrast, the establishment of a uniform, reliable and repeatable temperature pattern across the back, neck, shoulders, chest and croup is difficult due to the presence of muscle tissue, which undergoes varying degrees of physiological change depending on the level and type of exercise or performance.

The following sections present examples of body surface temperature distribution for selected body areas of healthy horses undergoing regular training.

3.2.3.2 Back area

A thermogram of the back area includes the thoracic and lumbar vertebrae. Muscles running along this area give stability, support and mobility to the spine. These muscles include the longissimus dorsi muscle, the iliocostalis dorsi muscle and the spinalis dorsi muscle, the most important of which is the longissimus dorsi (Haussler *et al.*, 2001; Peham *et al.*, 2010). This muscle acts to stabilize the spine during movement. The supraspinous ligament is attached

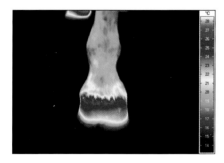

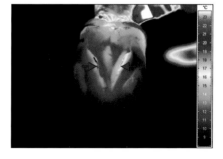

Fig. 3.12. Thermogram of the right forelimb hoof from the dorsal aspect. The highest surface temperature is found in the coronary band. The surface temperature of the hoof becomes gradually cooler towards the ground.

Fig. 3.13. Thermogram of the hoof sole of the right forelimb from the solar aspect, showing an equal surface temperature on the sole, frog and heel. The highest surface temperature is in both hoof bars (red arrows).

to the poll area and connects the spinous processes of the thoracic and lumbar vertebrae, contributing to spine stabilization (Figs 3.14 and 3.15).

In the healthy horse, the surface temperature map of the back has a uniform distribution, both on the spine and laterally on either side of the spine (Figs 3.16 and 3.17).

In riding horses, the muscles, tendons and ligaments of the spine are subjected to a variety of loads. Constant training loads the back musculoskeletal system, increasing its blood circulation. In such cases, the surface body

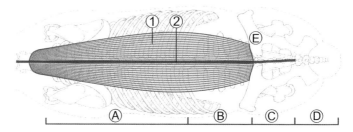

Fig. 3.14. Back area from the dorsal aspect with the thoracic vertebrae (A), lumbar vertebrae (B), sacral vertebrae (C), coccygeal vertebrae (D), pelvis (E), longissimus dorsi muscle (1) and supraspinous ligament (2) indicated.

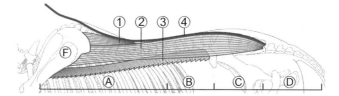

Fig. 3.15. Back area from the lateral aspect with the thoracic vertebrae (A), lumbar vertebrae (B), sacral vertebrae (C), coccygeal vertebrae (D), scapula (F), spinalis dorsi muscle (1), longissimus dorsi muscle (2), iliocostalis dorsi muscle (3) and supraspinous ligament (4) identified.

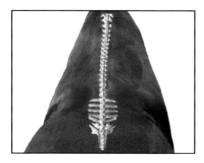

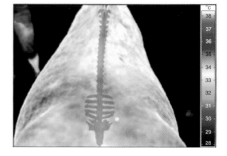

Fig. 3.16. Dorsal aspect of the back with the thoracolumbar vertebrae indicated.

Fig. 3.17. Thermogram of the back from the dorsal aspect with the thoracolumbar vertebrae indicated.

temperature along the midline of the spine of a horse at rest can be up to 2–3°C higher at the thoracic and lumbar vertebrae than seen laterally on either side of the back (von Schweinitz, 1999; Tunley and Henson, 2004).

Research carried out on racehorses has indicated that the warmest part of the spine is at the thoracic vertebrae (Soroko *et al.*, 2012). The elevated temperature of this part of the spine could be the result of intensive performance in the case of a racehorse or could be due to rider imbalance, an incorrectly fitted saddle and/or poor riding technique. Peham *et al.* (2010) demonstrated that the highest load (expressed in Newtons (N)) on the horse's back is encountered during a sitting trot (2112 N), followed by a rising trot (2056 N) and the two-point seat jumping position (1688 N). Hence any rider imbalance, especially at a sitting trot, is likely to cause asymmetry in, or an elevated, temperature.

3.2.3.3 Shoulder area

A thermogram of the shoulder area from the lateral aspect includes the area of the withers, the base of the neck, the shoulder and the elbow joints. Muscles around the shoulder are responsible for motion of the shoulder and elbow joints. The main muscle responsible for both flexion of the shoulder joint and extension of the elbow joint is the triceps brachii muscle. This muscle extends between the shoulder and the humerus bone. The muscle responsible for extension of the shoulder joint and for flexion of the elbow joint is the biceps brachii muscle (Fig. 3.18).

The shoulder area has cold spots around the shoulder and elbow joints, as the joint fluid lowers the temperature compared with the surrounding soft tissues. The base of the neck is warm due to the heat accumulation characteristic

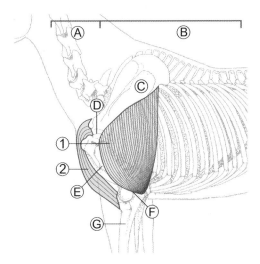

Fig. 3.18. Left shoulder from the lateral aspect with the cervical vertebrae (A), thoracic vertebrae (B), scapula (C), shoulder joint (D), humerus (E), elbow joint (F), radius (G), triceps brachii muscle (1) and biceps brachii muscle (2) indicated.

of concave surfaces of the body. Similarly, the area behind the elbow joint has a higher body surface temperature (Figs 3.19 and 3.20).

3.2.3.4 *Neck area*

A thermogram of the neck area from the lateral aspect should include the area from the base of the neck to the poll. Muscles above the cervical vertebrae area are responsible for lifting and bending of the neck. The main muscle responsible for neck extension and side movements is the splenius muscle. This fills most of the neck and runs along the cervical vertebrae to the withers area. The rhomboid muscle runs along the top of the neck under the mane, with connection to the nuchal ligament and insertion in the medial scapular cartilage. The function of this muscle is to elevate the neck and draw the scapula forwards and upwards (Fig. 3.21).

    The neck area is characterized by a higher body surface temperature along the jugular groove, where the jugular veins are superficially located. The other

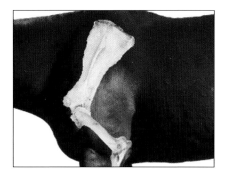

Fig. 3.19. Left shoulder from the lateral aspect with the scapula, humerus, shoulder joint and elbow joint indicated.

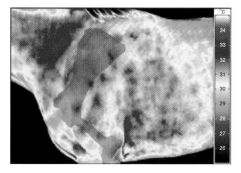

Fig. 3.20. Thermogram of the left shoulder from the lateral aspect with the scapula, humerus, shoulder joint and elbow joint indicated.

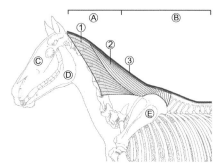

Fig. 3.21. Left side of the neck from the lateral aspect with the cervical vertebrae (A), thoracic vertebrae (B), maxilla (upper jaw; C), mandible (lower jaw; D), scapula (E), splenius muscle (1), rhomboid muscle (2) and nuchal ligament (3) indicated.

parts of the neck area are characterized by uniform temperature distribution. Sometimes the upper part of the neck, just under the mane, can have a lower surface temperature due to accumulated fatty tissue (Figs 3.22 and 3.23).

3.2.3.5 Head area

A thermogram of the head area from the lateral aspect should include the whole lateral aspect of the head plus the ears. The largest muscle of the head is the masseter muscle and is the primary muscle for chewing. The main function of the muscle is to bring the upper jaw and lower jaw together and to move the bottom jaw from side to side. The next major muscle is the temporalis muscle, the function of which is to close the mandible (Fig. 3.24).

The thermographic pattern of the lateral aspect of the head shows that the eyes and nostrils are equally the warmest areas. The temporomandibular area has lower surface temperature compared with the surrounding area (Figs 3.25 and 3.26).

3.2.3.6 Croup area

A thermogram of the croup area from the lateral aspect includes the flank, the lumbar and coccygeal vertebrae, and the stifle joint. From the dorsal aspect, the area includes the sacroiliac joints, the sacral vertebrae, the pelvis (including the tuber coxae) and the dock area. From the caudal aspect, the area includes the body area between the dock and the stifle joint. The main muscle at the croup from the lateral aspect is the quadriceps femoris muscle, which fills the space between the hip joint and the stifle joint and is responsible, along with other muscles, for flexing the stifle joint (Fig. 3.27). The muscles from the dorsal aspect are the gluteal group muscles, responsible for extension and flexion of the hip joint (Fig. 3.28). The muscles from the caudal aspect are the biceps femoris muscle, and the semitendinosus and semimembranosus muscles, responsible for extension of the hip joint (Fig. 3.29).

The lateral aspect of the croup has the warmest areas around the flank due to the shorter and thinner hair coat in this area. The area between the

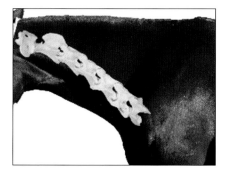

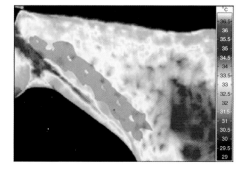

Fig. 3.22. Left side of the neck from the lateral aspect with the cervical vertebrae indicated.

Fig. 3.23. Thermogram of the left side of the neck from the lateral aspect with the cervical vertebrae indicated, with the warmer jugular groove area below.

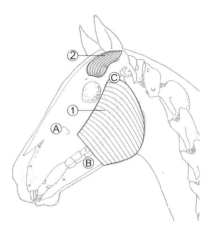

Fig. 3.24. Skull (head) from the left lateral aspect with the maxilla (upper jaw; A), mandible (lower jaw; B), temporomandibular joint (C), masseter muscle (1) and temporalis muscle (2) indicated.

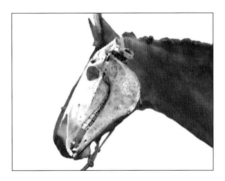

Fig. 3.25. Left side of the head from the lateral aspect with the skull indicated.

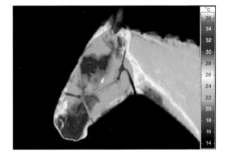

Fig. 3.26. Thermogram of the left side of the head from the lateral aspect with the skull indicated.

pelvis, hip joint and stifle joint has a higher surface temperature compared with other areas of the croup, which are more exposed to the environment. The stifle joint has a comparatively lower temperature due to accumulated joint fluid (Fig. 3.30 and 3.31).

The dorsal aspect of the croup has a symmetrical temperature distribution on either side of the spine (Figs 3.32 and 3.33).

The caudal aspect of the croup has the warmest areas along the semimembranosus muscles running along the tail (Figs 3.34 and 3.35).

3.2.3.7   Chest area

A thermogram of the chest area from the lateral aspect includes the back area (thoracic and lumbar vertebrae) and the lower part of the barrel including the flank and the elbow joint area. The muscles of the chest area include the rectus abdominis muscle, which is responsible for flexing and supporting the spine. The obliquus externus abdominis and obliquus internus abdominis muscles flex the spine, support the chest area and compress the abdominal viscera (Fig. 3.36).

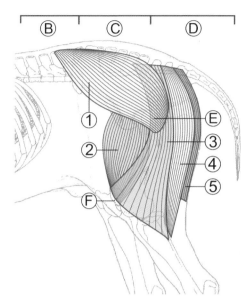

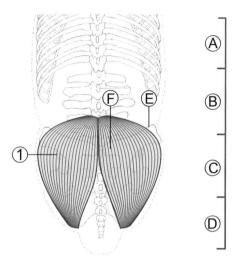

Fig. 3.27. Left croup from the lateral aspect with the lumbar vertebrae (B), sacral vertebrae (C), coccygeal vertebrae (D), hip joint (E), stifle joint (F), gluteal group muscles (1), quadriceps femoris muscle (2), biceps femoris muscle (3), semitendinosus muscle (4) and semimembranosus muscle (5) indicated.

Fig. 3.28. Croup from the dorsal aspect with the thoracic vertebrae (A), lumbar vertebrae (B), sacral vertebrae (C), coccygeal vertebrae (D), pelvis (E), sacroiliac joint (F) and gluteal group muscles (1) indicated.

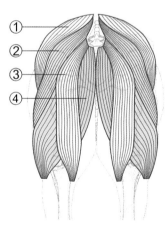

Fig. 3.29. Croup from the caudal aspect with the gluteal group muscles (1), biceps femoris muscle (2), semitendinosus muscle (3) and semimembranosus muscle (4) indicated.

The chest area to the barrel has a uniform temperature distribution, with the flank area, and the area behind the elbow joint having a comparatively higher body surface temperature (Figs 3.37 and 3.38).

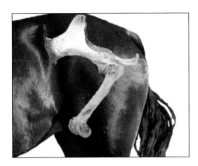

Fig. 3.30. Left croup from the lateral aspect with the pelvis, femur and hip joint indicated.

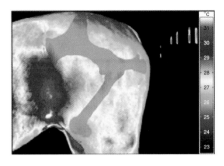

Fig. 3.31. Thermogram of the left croup from the lateral aspect with the pelvis, femur and hip joint indicated.

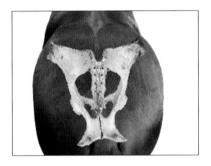

Fig. 3.32. Croup from the dorsal aspect with the pelvis and sacrum indicated.

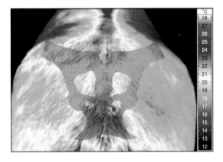

Fig. 3.33. Thermogram of the croup from the dorsal aspect with the pelvis and sacrum indicated.

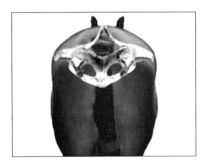

Fig. 3.34. Croup from the caudal aspect with the pelvis indicated.

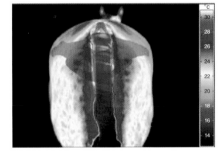

Fig. 3.35. Thermogram of the croup from the caudal aspect with the pelvis indicated.

3.2.4   What should be considered in thermographic image interpretation?

Thermography enables abnormal patterns in skin body surface temperatures (and hence vascularity and metabolic activity within and below the skin surface) to be detected (Turner, 1991). Variation in skin temperature is due to changes

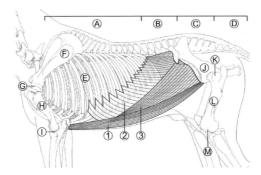

Fig. 3.36. Left side of the chest from the lateral aspect with the thoracic vertebrae (A), lumbar vertebrae (B), sacral vertebrae (C), coccygeal vertebrae (D), ribs (E), scapula (F), shoulder joint (G), humerus (H), elbow joint (I), pelvis (J), hip joint (K), femur (L), stifle joint (M), rectus abdominis muscle (1), obliquus externus abdominis muscle (2) and obliquus internus abdominis muscle (3) indicated.

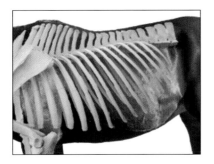

Fig. 3.37. Left side of the chest from the lateral aspect with the thoracolumbar vertebrae and rib cage indicated.

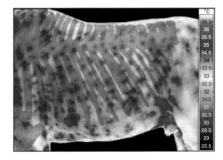

Fig. 3.38. Thermogram of the left side of the chest from the lateral aspect with the thoracolumbar vertebrae and rib cage indicated.

in the local blood circulation associated with inflammation, and is recognized thermographically as 'hotspots' (Ring, 1990; Turner, 2001). Other pathological conditions reduce blood circulation due to vascular shunts, thrombosis or autonomic nervous system abnormalities, and are recognized as 'coldspots' (Turner, 1991; von Schweinitz, 1999).

Inflammation can occur in different stages: subclinical (early), clinical (apparent) and chronic (persistent). For each stage, the intensity of vascularization will be different. Examples of local inflammation at three different stages are presented in Figs 3.39–3.41. Subclinical inflammation (Fig. 3.39) shows increased vascularization only in the injured area. Clinical inflammation (Fig 3.40) is characterized by increased vascularization spreading around the injury. However, chronic inflammation (Fig. 3.41), similar to subclinical inflammation, shows increased vascularization only in the injured area.

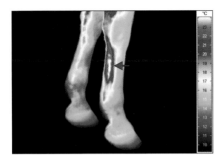
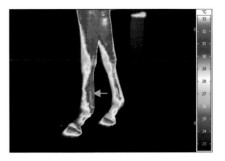

Fig. 3.39. Thermogram of the distal right
and left forelimbs from the lateral and
medial aspects, respectively. Subclinical
inflammation of the right forelimb is
indicated (red arrow).

Fig. 3.40. Thermogram of the distal left
and right forelimbs from the lateral and
medial aspects, respectively. Clinical
inflammation of the left forelimb is
indicated (green arrow).

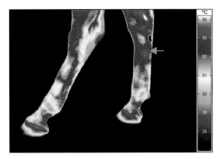

Fig. 3.41. Thermogram of the distal left and right hindlimbs from the lateral
and medial aspects, respectively. Chronic inflammation in the right hindlimb
is indicated (green arrow).

Inflammation occurring in the distal limbs may sometimes be confused
with training overload effects. Training overloads often result in greater vascularization of the distal limbs, which does not necessarily cause inflammation but can be an adaptive change. An asymmetric limb load, however,
may be associated with a compensation effect. This happens when an injury occurs in one limb, and the opposite limb works harder to reduce
the load on the injured side. This results in stronger vascularization of the
healthy limb (especially around the joints) and thus an increase in its surface temperature.

It should also be considered that decreased surface temperature can be
associated with thrombosis, swelling that results in decreased circulation in
damaged tissue or the presence of dense scar tissue. An area with a locally
reduced body surface temperature may also be caused by a neurological disorder. The cutaneous vasculature is regulated by the sympathetic nervous
system. A functional disorder of one of the nerves in the neck, thoracic or
lumbar vertebrae can contribute to skin vascularization changes in the area

controlled by that nerve. A summary skin nerve map of the forelimbs and hindlimbs of a horse is presented in Figs 3.42 and 3.43. Vertebrae displacement can also result in nerve cord compression, reducing the vascularization of the skin in a location remote from the area controlled by the affected nerve. Therefore, observing a body surface temperature decrease in a specific area that is controlled by a relevant nerve may indicate a neurological problem in a specific area of the spine.

Nerve compression or inflammation may also result in a temperature decrease at the site of injury. However, preventing nerve conduction by the use of chemical or surgical nerve blocks results in increased body surface temperature in the area controlled by this nerve (Purohit, 2008).

3.2.5 Thermographic reports

The final stage of thermogram interpretation is the production of a thermographic report. The report should include the data from the owner questionnaire (see Chapter 2, this volume) containing basic information about the horse, details of the environmental conditions and the preparation of the horse for the examination, as well as thermographic analysis and conclusions.

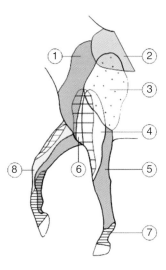

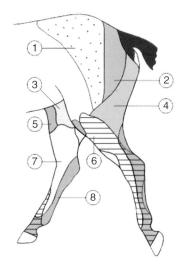

Fig. 3.42. Cutaneous innervation of the forelimb with the supraclavicular nerve (1), dorsolateral branch of the thoracic nerve (2), intercostobrachial nerve (3), radial nerve (4), ulnar nerve (5), axillary nerve (6), median nerve (7) and musculocutaneous nerve (8) indicated.

Fig. 3.43. Cutaneous innervation of the hindlimb with the cranial cluneal nerve (1), middle cluneal nerve (2), genitofemoral nerve (3), caudal cutaneous femoral nerve (4), lateral cutaneous femoral nerve (5), peroneal nerve (6), saphenous nerve (7) and tibial nerve (8) indicated.

The report should consist of five parts:

- **Part 1**: information about the horse (name, age, breed), plus data about the owner and the stable.
- **Part 2**: explanation of the purpose of the thermographic examination and the horse's characteristics, its current state of health and any factors that may have contributed to the problems currently being experienced by the horse (e.g. poor conformation, saddle-fit issues, type of training).
- **Part 3**: a description of the thermographic examination conditions, including date, time of the examination and the environmental conditions in the room, and a description of the horse's preparation for the examination.
- **Part 4**: presentation of labelled and numbered thermograms with relevant comments.
- **Part 5**: summary and conclusions drawn from the thermograms.

In the interpretation of the thermograms, a knowledge of body surface temperature symmetry and repeatability of the temperature maps, combined with an understanding of temperature ranges in the healthy horse and the effect of environment, training, past and present injuries, etc. is essential. This knowledge can then be related to the anatomy and physiological condition of the animal. Therefore, in some cases, interpretation of thermograms based only on body surface temperature distribution may be misleading or unclear. The correct interpretation of thermograms must be based not only on the images themselves but also on the interview with the horse owner or trainer and the horse's current problems, as well as present and past injuries, the environment, etc.

A knowledge and understanding of the following are required by the thermographic practitioner in order to draw accurate and meaningful conclusions from thermographic images taken:

- Infrared radiation emission (establishing the appropriate measurement conditions).
- Functioning of the thermographic camera and software for correct image interpretation.
- The main bone and muscle structures of the horse, especially in the areas of the neck, shoulders, chest and croup.
- The anatomy of the distal limbs, including the tendons, ligaments and blood vessels.
- The temperature distribution across the healthy horse at low and high ambient temperatures.
- The effect that environmental factors may have on the body surface temperature measurements.

4

Development of Equine Thermography and its Use in Equestrianism

4.1 Development of Thermography in Equine Veterinary Medicine

In the early 1970s, thermography began to be used as a diagnostic tool, complementary to standard radiographic and ultrasonographic examinations in veterinary medicine. Most of the publications of this period were presented by Strömberg (1971, 1972, 1974), where the first results of thermographic examinations in the detection and monitoring of injuries of distal limbs of racehorses were described. It was demonstrated that subclinical inflammation of the superficial digital flexor tendon could be detected up to 14 days before the appearance of clinical signs of inflammation. Thermographic examination detected an increased temperature in the injured limb, despite radiography failing to indicate any pathological changes. The early detection of inflammation gives thermography a unique value in sport horse veterinary diagnosis. Early injury detection or prediction, through identification of areas of weakness, brings with it the opportunity to protect the horse from more serious injury by applying early treatment.

In the 1980s, the use of thermography in the diagnosis of orthopaedic injuries was investigated by Purohit and McCoy (1980). They used thermography of the splint bone area to demonstrate the effectiveness of anti-inflammatory drugs. Thermographic images confirmed the reduction of inflammation in response to treatment. However, when no heat was detected by manual palpation of the affected area, thermography continued to suggest increased blood circulation and hence incomplete recovery. In the same study, thermography was compared with radiographic examination in the detection of subluxation of the third lumbar vertebrae. The resulting large mass of soft tissue meant that radiographic images were unable to detect the site of injury, whereas thermography was effective in identification of the exact site of the pathology. Thermography was also effective in localizing hoof abscesses, laminitis, tendonitis and stifle

© M. Soroko and M.C.G. Davies Morel 2016. *Equine Thermography in Practice*
(M. Soroko and M.C.G. Davies Morel)

joint inflammation. Further research by the same authors focused on the application of thermography in the diagnosis of Horner's syndrome, a neurological disease involving nerve paralysis of the sympathetic nervous system around the head and neck. The affected area showed a local increase in body surface temperature of 2–3°C due to vasodilation. Thermography was therefore demonstrated to be potentially very useful in the diagnosis and treatment of the disease (Purohit et al., 1980). Similarly, at this time thermography also proved to be useful in the diagnosis of tarsal joint inflammation. Work by Vaden et al. (1980) examined 20 racehorses. One horse presented with clinical signs of tarsal joint inflammation, which was confirmed by thermographic and radiographic examinations. Another four presented with abnormal blood circulation changes around the tarsal joint on thermography, although radiography did not detect any signs or lesions. The study indicated that thermography, along with radiography, can be a useful tool for the diagnosis of chronic tarsal joint inflammation, particularly in the early stages of joint disorders when no changes are detected in radiographic examinations. Similar conclusions were drawn by Bowman et al. (1983), who demonstrated the use of thermography in detecting subclinical inflammation of the tarsal and carpal joints and in monitoring recovery after intra-joint corticosteroid injection. Interestingly, it appeared that corticosteroid treatment of the tarsal joint accelerated recovery, whereas this was not evident in the carpal joint.

Navicular syndrome was another area of investigation, with affected horses reported as presenting with a lack of temperature increase in the affected limb after exercise. The thermographic results correlated with radiography findings, which showed an increased vascular foramina of the affected navicular bone and hence decreased blood flow and cooler surface temperatures. It was therefore suggested that thermography could be used to recognize navicular syndrome in the early stages (Turner et al., 1983).

The 1990s saw research focus on the potential of thermography in monitoring drug efficacy. Ghafir et al. (1996) used thermography to monitor treatment of, rather than just diagnose, Horner's syndrome. Temperature measurements of the head area were performed before and 30 min after an α2-adrenoreceptor agonist injection was given to two horses with clinical signs of the disease. After drug administration, the head surface temperature measurements showed a temperature decrease, thus confirming the effectiveness of the drug.

Thermographic examinations were also demonstrated to be useful in diagnosing not only distal limb abnormalities (laminitis, stress fractures, sole abscesses and tendonitis) but also upper limb (above the tarsal and carpal joints) abnormalities (muscle strain and inflammation, croup and caudal thigh myopathies, and general neuromuscular disease; Turner, 1991, 1996). Turner (1996) used thermography to detect inflammation in three areas of the upper hindlimb: the cranial thigh, caudal thigh and croup region. Inflammation in the cranial thigh appeared as hotspots associated with the quadriceps proximal to the insertion of the patella. In the caudal thigh, the most common area of inflammation was the musculotendinous junction of the semitendinosus muscle and biceps femoris. Inflammation was also visualized in the croup region over the third trochanter, sacroiliac region and gluteus muscle and over the loin region.

In a later study, Turner (1998) used thermography to detect inflammation of muscles in the forelimbs, including the pectoralis muscles and biceps brachialis muscles. In a study of horses with croup or caudal thigh myopathy, 20 of 23 horses with palpable areas of pain had corresponding abnormal areas visualized by thermography. Therefore, thermography was recommended as a tool for detecting upper-limb lameness, by confirming inflammation of sore areas requiring further diagnostics. A further study by Kold and Chappell (1998) investigated the effectiveness of thermography in detecting inflammation along the spine in the acute stage. Thermography effectively identified increased activity of the superficial soft tissue of the thoracic spine and symmetrically over the sacroiliac area.

Once abnormalities have been detected and confirmed, thermography can also be used to determine the effectiveness of different types of therapeutic and rehabilitation interventions (Turner, 1996, 1998), including the effectiveness of acupuncture therapy in neuromuscular disease (von Schweinitz, 1998).

Further work by von Schweinitz (1999) demonstrated thermography to be the most sensitive method for diagnosing subclinical and chronic back conditions, particularly neuromuscular diseases of the thoracolumbar spine. The inflamed spine areas present with an increased body surface temperature.

In the 2000s, the regular use of thermography in racehorse lameness during training was investigated. One particular study monitored 45 horses over 1 year using regular thermographic examinations of the distal limbs. During the examinations, nine of the horses had clinical and chronic inflammation diagnosed, causing them to be withdrawn from racing. In all cases, subclinical inflammation was detected by thermography at least 2 weeks before it became clinically evident. This indicated the potential of thermography in regularly monitoring distal limbs to detect early-stage inflammation and help to avoid future clinical conditions and loss of soundness (Turner *et al.*, 2001). Similarly, thermography was demonstrated to be an effective complementary tool in the diagnosis of thoracic and lumbar vertebrae problems (Fonseca *et al.*, 2006). Thermography was used to identify the area of injury, and ultrasonography was then used to ascertain the type of injury. Such complementary use of thermography along with ultrasonography was demonstrated to be efficient at detecting supraspinous and interspinous ligament inflammation, dorsal intervertebral osteoarthritis and kissing spines of the thoracolumbar spine (Fonseca *et al.*, 2006). Work by Levet *et al.* (2009) used thermography to monitor the superficial and deep dermal sores that may result from leg plaster casts for fractured distal limbs. This allowed optimum timing for plaster cast removal to be determined and the avoidance of serious complications leading to prolonged wound care.

From 2010 onwards, the regular use of thermographic examination to monitor and potentially predict injuries was increasingly investigated. Soroko (2011a) reported on the regular examination of the distal limbs of racehorses during the racing season, identifying areas of past injury and the effect of training loads. This proved helpful in managing and monitoring treatments and training programmes. These regular examinations enabled the diagnosis of an early-stage dorsal metacarpal disease (known as bucked shins) (Soroko, 2011b; Figs 4.1 and 4.2). In the racing industry, approximately 70% of young

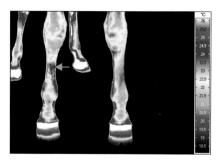

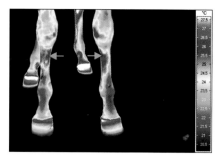

Fig. 4.1. Thermogram of the distal right and left forelimbs from the dorsal aspect. Subclinical inflammation of the right third metacarpal bone is indicated (green arrow).

Fig. 4.2. Thermogram of the distal right and left forelimbs from the dorsal aspect. Clinical inflammation of the right and left third metacarpal bones is indicated (green arrows).

Thoroughbreds are diagnosed with bucked shins. This condition affects young horses, resulting in temporary withdrawal from, and disruption to, their vital early phase of training (Katayama *et al.*, 2001).

Currently, thermography is used in veterinary medicine as a complementary tool in the diagnosis of a variety of limb injuries including hoof abscesses, laminitis, tendonitis, inflammation of the fetlock joint, and carpal and tarsal joint inflammation (Figs 4.3–4.6). For back abnormalities, thermography has been successfully applied to study muscular and spinous process inflammation of the thoracic vertebrae and disorders of the sacroiliac joint (Figs 4.7–4.9).

The numerous publications available on the applications of thermography in veterinary medicine have proved its advantages in diagnosing abnormalities and its ability to detect the early signs of inflammation of the musculoskeletal system in sport horses. As a result, scientific and rehabilitation centres specializing in thermographic diagnosis of horses have been established. Their research is focused primarily on the monitoring of anti-inflammatory drug effectiveness and recovery from neurological disease, as well as diagnosing diseases of the back and limbs (Purohit *et al.*, 2004; Purohit, 2008). However, other studies have moved towards internal body temperature estimation by, for example, measuring the surface temperature around the corner of the horse's eye. This is reported to be useful in non-invasive temperature monitoring for fever (Johnson *et al.*, 2011). Further work has investigated the use of thermography in the welfare evaluation of horses. Fleischmann *et al.* (2009) reported a different temperature distribution pattern across the head of healthy horses compared with those showing symptoms of pain. Variations in skin temperature caused by peripheral vasoconstriction have been reported to depend on the physiological and emotional stress of the horse. The results obtained by Valera *et al.* (2012) indicated that thermography is an efficient method for detecting stress in horses subjected to the acute events in, for example, show jumping; body surface temperature measurements correlating with salivary cortisol measurements. More recently, a study by McGreevy *et al.* (2012) suggested that horses wearing double bridles and tight nosebands, which restrict

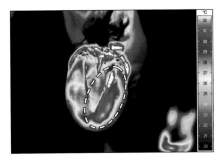

Fig. 4.3. Thermogram of the left hoof sole from the solar aspect. An abscess in the medial aspect of the hoof sole is indicated (dashed outline).

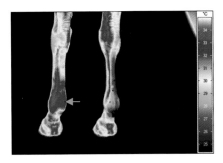

Fig. 4.4. Thermogram of the distal part of the left and right forelimbs from palmar aspect. Inflammation of the superficial digital flexor tendon of the left forelimb is indicated (green arrow).

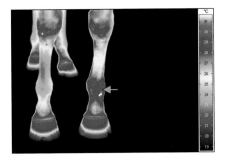

Fig. 4.5. Thermogram of the distal right and left forelimbs from the dorsal aspect. Inflammation of the fetlock joint of the left forelimb is indicated (green arrow).

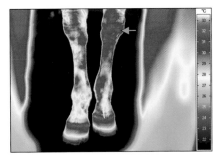

Fig. 4.6. Thermogram of the distal right and left hindlimbs from the dorsal aspect. Inflammation of the tarsal joint of the left hindlimb is indicated (green arrow).

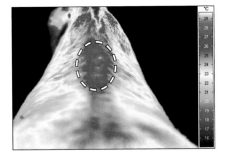

Fig. 4.7. Thermogram of the back from the dorsal aspect illustrating an increased body surface temperature indicative of inflammation of the spinous processes of the thoracic vertebrae (dashed outline).

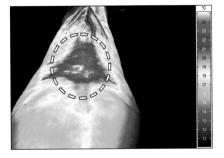

Fig. 4.8. Thermogram of the back from the dorsal aspect illustrating an increase in body surface temperature indicative of inflammation of the back muscles in the thoracic vertebrae area (dashed outline).

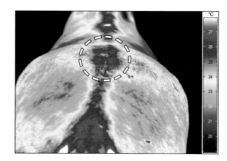

Fig. 4.9. Thermogram of the croup from the dorsal aspect. Inflammation of the sacroiliac joints. Area marked with a dashed outline.

jaw movements, had an increased eye temperature, suggesting a physiological stress response (see section 4.2.1).

Finally, thermography has been used in the assessment of sporting performance in racehorses (Soroko *et al.*, 2014, 2015; see section 4.3).

4.2 Use of Thermography in Equestrianism

Many areas of equestrianism employ thermography to assist in the management and training of horses in order to ensure optimum performance but not at the expense of welfare.

4.2.1 Use of thermography to monitor horse welfare

Since 2009, thermography has been considered to be a potential diagnostic method by the International Equestrian Federation (FEI). For more than 90 years, the FEI has promoted equestrianism in all its forms and has encouraged the development of the FEI disciplines, setting rules and regulations throughout the world. One of the core values of the FEI is promoting respect for, and the welfare of, horses involved in international equestrian sports. For this purpose, the FEI has developed welfare regulations to ensure that the entire equine community – athletes, veterinarians, grooms, managers, coaches, owners and officials – help combat doping and the inappropriate use of medications through better education and increased vigilance at each stage of a horse's preparation for a particular discipline. One example of horse welfare infringement is the artificial irritation of the skin of the limbs, by chemical application to the distal limbs, causing hypersensitivity. The goal is to encourage horses to jump over the fences higher and more carefully to prevent the pain caused by touching an obstacle. Hypersensitivity to touch is related to a local increase in tissue blood circulation (and thus increased body surface temperature). Hence, the FEI introduced thermography as a permitted complementary diagnostic method for easier detection of artificially induced temperature changes in the limbs of jumping horses. The capacity for non-invasive assessment of the inflammation stage qualifies thermography as a safe tool to detect such use of illegal chemicals.

In order to detect any possible limb skin irritation, examining veterinarians may perform thermographic examinations but only in connection with clinical examination. During the Olympic Games in 1996, thermography proved an effective tool in detecting limb irritation in jumping horses. Today, it is an FEI officially approved tool to aid in the diagnosis of increased limb sensitivity during Concours de Saint International (CSI)-level competitions.

Studies on the application of thermography for the detection of the use of chemical agents on, and mechanical damage to, performance horses began in the 1970s (Stephan and Gorlach, 1971; Nelson and Osheim, 1975). Thermography has also proved useful in detecting illegal procedures in show horses, such as detecting the application of irritants to the perineal region to enhance tail elevation. The goal of this procedure is to lift the tail in order to improve the horse's presentation. In some breeds (e.g. Arab), this is a very important feature in conformation evaluation. As a result of the irritating agent, the perineal region shows an elevated temperature, visible on thermograms (Turner and Scoggins, 1985).

Thermography has also been used to investigate the practice of applying inflammatory counter-irritants topically (e.g. 10% mercuric iodide) or injected subdermally (e.g. isopropyl alcohol), and induction of hypersensitization using limb bandages containing metallic objects. Van Hoogmoed et al. (2000) used chemical-irritants applied to the dorsal aspect of the pastern, and metallic irritants contained in limb bandages to the metacarpal area to induce hypersensitivity of that area. Thermographic images detected changed thermal patterns for 6 days after a single topical application of mercuric iodide. In the case of subdermal isopropyl alcohol injection, the elevated temperature was observed to last for 8 days, and after the use of metallic bottle caps within leg wraps, an elevated temperature was detected for 24 h.

Standard thermographic examination methods to diagnose hypersensitivity of the limbs appear in Annex XI of the FEI Veterinary Regulations (the 'Annex XI Protocol' 2012). These regulations contain a detailed thermographic examination protocol together with required clinical examinations using palpation and observation during CSI competitions. They provide the following information:

* Thermography is one of the complementary diagnostic tools used for confirmation of the application of skin-irritating chemicals.
* The limb examination of a horse may be performed before, or immediately after, competition by a designated FEI veterinarian, and only in a stable.
* All thermographic examinations must be carried out in a controlled environment.
* The thermographic examination should include the forelimbs from the dorsal aspect from carpal joints to hooves, and the hindlimbs from the dorsal aspect from tarsal joints to hooves. The goal of the thermographic examination is to detect invalid heat patterns on the surface of the limbs. The horse also has a clinical examination, based on palpation (manual pressure) and

observation. All examinations are performed simultaneously by two examining veterinarians.

- In the case that the thermographic examination reveals differences between symmetrical limbs exceeding 2°C, or in the case that both limbs show very high or very low temperature and, in addition, the horse presents with incorrect responses to pressure during the palpation examination, then the horse can be eliminated from competition. The case must be submitted to the Grand Jury and the Veterinary Delegate to decide whether the horse should be allowed to continue in the competition or be disqualified.

Horses with hypersensitive limbs may be disqualified on the basis of horse welfare and fair play. However, limb hypersensitivity is not always the result of chemical application; it can be produced by a range of normal occurrences such as insect stings, accidental self-inflicted injuries and skin infections. Hyposensitivity could result from traumatic or surgical cutting of the nerves in that area of the limb (i.e. neurectomy). For this reason, thermographic examination combined with clinical examination is the first and decisive step before taking a horse for further investigation. Any horse disqualified due to hypersensitivity must go through Anti-Doping control (Equine Anti-Doping and Controlled Medication Regulations). According to FEI General Regulations (Article 159.6 FEI.2, 1596.4), there is no appeal against the decision of the Grand Jury, following a final examination, to disqualify a horse for abnormal limb sensitivity.

4.2.2   Use of thermography to assess saddle fit

Thermography can also be used to aid the correct fit of the saddle to the horse's back. Tack-related problems can be identified by the thermal patterns caused by the tack while the horse is being ridden. For proper saddle-fit assessment, two thermographic examinations should be performed of a horse's back: at rest and immediately after exercise. The body temperature distribution of the back before training confirms any potential injuries. After the first examination, the horse should be tacked up with a single numnah and exercised for a minimum of 20 min. The second examination of the horse's back is performed immediately after untacking the horse. Thermographic examination indicates the temperature distribution, and thus the interaction between the saddle and the back muscles. This pressure distribution should be the same on both sides of the spine (Fig. 4.10). Locally warmer areas on the back indicate higher saddle pressure. Conversely, locally cooler areas indicate less saddle contact with the back. 'Bridging' is the most common reason for an improper saddle fit. A bridging saddle has a greater interaction on the back at two points: at the level of the pommel and of the cantle on both sides of the back (Fig. 4.11). Saddle asymmetry is also a significant problem that can be identified through thermography. Work in Brazil evaluated 62 saddles used on 129 jumping horses. Thermograms of each horse's back and saddle were performed after training. The images obtained allowed evaluation of a range of features including contact between the saddle and spine, asymmetry in the area of interaction between the saddle panels and the back of the horse, and asymmetry between the panels.

The saddles had direct contact with the spine in 37.2% of horses, while 55.8% demonstrated asymmetry in the image of the back (Fig. 4.12) and asymmetry between the saddle panels was evident in 62.8% of cases (Fig. 4.13) (Arruda *et al.*, 2011). Despite being a useful tool for saddle fitting, it must be remembered that there are many external factors that influence the final thermographic image. Therefore, interpretation of the thermogram requires careful consideration.

4.2.3   Use of thermography to assess hoof function

Thermography is also useful in the assessment of the balancing/function of hooves, both shod and unshod. When a horse with metal shoes is examined immediately after trotting on a hard surface, the part of the shoe covering the side of the hoof that is taking the greatest load appears warmer. Thermography

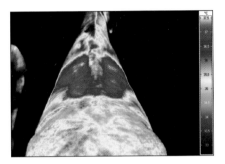

Fig. 4.10. Thermogram of the back from the dorsal aspect, taken 30 min after training in a dressage saddle. The back surface temperature distribution is equal on both sides of the spine. This is an example of a correct saddle fit.

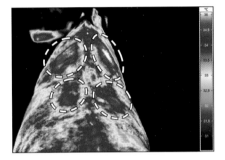

Fig. 4.11. Thermogram of the back from the dorsal aspect, taken 30 min after training in a jumping saddle. The pommel and cantle of the saddle put pressure on the back (dashed outlines). The middle part of the saddle seat has no contact with the back. This is an example of a bridging saddle.

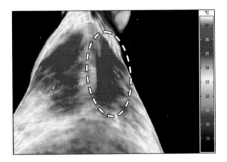

Fig. 4.12. Thermogram of the back from the dorsal aspect, taken 30 min after training in a jumping saddle. The saddle puts more pressure on the right side of the back (dashed outline).

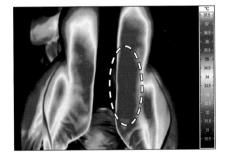

Fig. 4.13. Thermogram of jumping saddle panels taken 30 min after training. The right panel of the saddle puts more pressure on the back (dashed outline).

can also assess mediolateral hoof imbalance (Bathe, 2007). Thermographic images have demonstrated that the horseshoe can limit blood circulation in the main blood vessels of the distal limbs (Fig. 4.14). A horseshoe is a rigid element, which constrains the natural mechanics of working hooves, thus reducing the frog surface available for contact with the ground when the horse makes a step and restricting backflow of the blood from the hoof. A restricted blood flow reduces the nutrition and oxygen supply, resulting in poor hoof horn condition, as well as poorer regeneration of the tendons and joints, increasing susceptibility to injury. This is demonstrated in the case shown in Fig. 4.15, in which only one of the forelimbs is shod. When the shoe was removed, blood circulation in the limb was restored after 2 h (Fig. 4.16).

An example of an incorrectly functioning unshod hoof is illustrated in Figs 4.17 and 4.18, where the horse weight is distributed mostly on the side

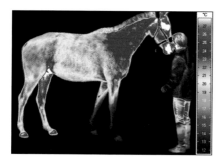

Fig. 4.14. Thermogram of the right side of the horse's body showing a decreased body surface temperature of the distal shod forelimbs and a normal body surface temperature of the distal part of the unshod hindlimbs.

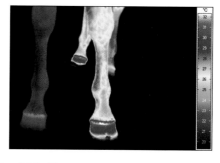

Fig. 4.15. Thermogram of the distal right and left forelimbs from the dorsal aspect showing normal body surface temperature distribution of the left unshod forelimb. In contrast, a decreased body surface temperature is evident in the right shod forelimb.

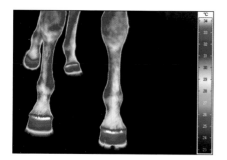

Fig. 4.16. Thermogram of the distal right and left forelimbs from the dorsal aspect. Two hours after the removal of the shoe from the right hoof, the distal right forelimb returned to a normal body surface temperature distribution.

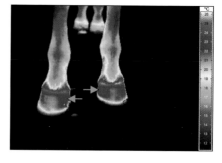

Fig. 4.17. Thermogram of the right and left front hooves from the dorsal aspect showing an increased surface temperature of both medial hoof walls compared with the lateral hoof walls (green arrows).

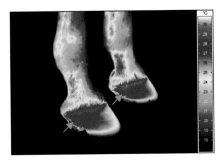

Fig. 4.18. Thermogram of the right and left front hooves from the lateral and medial aspects, respectively, showing an increased surface temperature of the lateral and medial walls of both hooves (blue arrows).

walls of the hooves. This would suggest a restricted function of the hoof, as well as incorrect operation of the tendons and ligaments in the distal limbs. This in turn adversely affects the muscles of the upper parts of the limb. The opposite situation should also be considered, when incorrect muscle function in the upper parts of the body result in defective function of the hooves.

4.3 Use of Thermography to Assess Racing Performance

Thermograms can be used to document the change in body surface temperature resulting from exercise and thus evaluate the function of individual parts of the body in sport and racing horses (Purohit and McCoy, 1980; Waldsmith and Oltmann, 1994; Jodkowska, 2005). Simon *et al.* (2006) highlighted the influence of exercise on body surface temperature of the forelimbs and hindlimbs. Thermal images of examined horses were taken before and after exercise on a treadmill. The body surface temperature overlying areas of muscle increased by 6°C after exercise, whereas the body surface temperature of the limbs increased by 8°C. There was a significant temperature rise during the first 15 min after exercise, which was no longer evident when thermographic examinations were performed 45 min after exercise. It was also found that muscular areas in the upper part of the body returned more quickly to the basal temperature than the distal limbs.

Jodkowska (2005) developed a model of horse body surface temperature before and after exercise and concluded that body surface temperature patterns were correlated with exercise performance. As such, body surface temperature examination of the distal limbs and back was helpful in assessing the quality of exercise and the preparation of the horse for training. It was also concluded that the optimum time for measuring body surface temperature was either before exercise or 24 h after exercise. Thermography can also be used as a valuable aid in the regular assessment of racehorses (Turner *et al.*, 2001). Thermographic imaging of the distal limbs and back at rest during the training season facilitated the detection of inflammation affecting performance (Soroko *et al.*, 2013).

Most notably, in the majority of cases, subclinical inflammation was detected 2 weeks before any clinical problems were noted. Not only training itself but also the type of training and performance influences body surface temperature distribution. For example, racehorses put more strain on the forelimbs, especially on the digital flexor tendons and bones. Regular thermographic examination of racehorses often found thermal abnormalities of the forelimbs associated with strains and overloads (Soroko, 2011a; Soroko *et al.*, 2014). This confirmed that racehorses are more likely to develop forelimb than hindlimb injuries (Peloso *et al.*, 1994). Work by Magnusson (1985) with 4-year-old Standardbred Trotters recorded increased injury in the left forelimb compared with the right, and concluded this was due to horses being raced and exercised on a clockwise race track; when resting, they were overloading the opposite side, resulting in the greater incidence of left limb injury. The opposite, however, was reported by Strömberg (1974) when horses trotted anti-clockwise at racing speed around a track with inadequately banked turns. This resulted in an increase in the left fetlock joint temperature of 0.4–2.2°C compared with the right limb.

Strains and overloading of the musculoskeletal system due to physical work result in increased blood circulation in a defensive adaptive process, predisposing the animal to future lameness (Evans *et al.*, 1992). High-intensity training and regular exercise can predispose horses to fatal skeletal injuries (Estberg *et al.*, 1995).

Increased body surface temperatures in the area of the back may also indicate pathological conditions caused by intensive performance in a horse, as well as rider imbalance or an incorrectly fitted saddle (Harman, 1999; De Cocq *et al.*, 2004; Arruda *et al.*, 2011). A reported 25% of horses in intensive training show injuries of the paraspinal muscles and ligaments (Jeffcott *et al.*, 1985). Other research has indicated body surface temperature variations in the sacroiliac joint region, a typical injury site for show-jumping horses with abnormalities of hindlimb movement (Haussler *et al.*, 1999). In racehorses under intensive training, the thoracic vertebrae had the highest body surface temperature when compared with the lumbar vertebrae and sacroiliac joint area (Soroko *et al.*, 2012). Higher body surface temperatures in the thoracic vertebrae are generally associated with riding, in particular at trot (Latif *et al.*, 2010). Compared with high-training intensity, gradual increments of exercise intensity over the long term caused less average body surface temperature differences between the thoracic vertebrae and the lumbar and sacroiliac joint areas when assessed at rest (Soroko *et al.*, 2012). In addition to the effects of training on the horse's back, regular thermographic examination of racehorses in training indicates an increased body surface temperature of the distal forelimbs at rest (Soroko *et al.*, 2015).

Finally, it is reported that the best-performing racehorses show a higher body surface temperature than their poorer-performing peers at all body sites at rest. Differences in temperature between the groups were significantly higher at the carpal joint, third metacarpal bone, fetlock joint, short pastern bone, tarsus joint (although only on the left side) and thoracic vertebrae (Soroko *et al.*, 2014). This temperature difference may reflect the increased physiological training impact and exertion during the race of the best-performing horses.

5 Use of Thermography in Physiotherapy

5.1 Thermography Applications in Equine Physiotherapy

The widest and most popular use of equine thermography is in physiotherapy. Animal physiotherapists use a range of treatments to try to improve the function of an animal's musculoskeletal system. The basic physiotherapy treatments include: massage, physiotherapy and kinesiotherapy. The use of massage treatment to reduce muscular pain and stimulate muscle development is particularly widespread (Sullivan *et al.*, 2005; Scott and Swenson, 2009). It is practised on racehorses and sport horses primarily to encourage recovery and regeneration after exercise, to improve flexibility and range of movement, and to promote full musculoskeletal system recovery after injury.

Musculoskeletal problems may be the result of cumulative disorders of soft tissue function (muscles, tendons and ligaments). A good example is muscle tension resulting from training overloads or because of incomplete recovery from chronic injuries. Sustained muscle tension over long periods reduces the horse's ability to use the full strength of the muscle, and may cause weakness over time. Increased muscle tension results in an unbalanced range of movement. In most cases, these problems cause gait abnormalities, decreased joint flexibility or stiffness on both sides of the body, and hence difficulties with lateral movements. The most common area where muscle tension appears is the back. Muscle spasms of the thoracic and lumbar vertebrae spread, through interlinked muscle chains, to other body areas causing disturbances in shoulder, neck, forelimb and hindlimb function. In many cases, this is related to poor saddle fit, poor conformation, previous injuries or an improper rider seat. Improper function of soft tissues is accompanied by changes in the cardiovascular system, which in turn result in temperature changes of both the affected and surrounding tissues, finally appearing as a change in body surface temperature. Thermography can be used to locate areas with altered temperature

© M. Soroko and M.C.G. Davies Morel 2016. *Equine Thermography in Practice* (M. Soroko and M.C.G. Davies Morel)

patterns, guiding the equine physiotherapist to concentrate on specific body sites during the rehabilitation process.

Case studies of two horses with muscle tension and one with flexor tendon overload are presented below.

CASE 1: MUSCLE TENSION OF THE BACK   This horse was a 5-year-old Polish Halfbred mare, and presented with back pain during grooming and tacking up. During exercise, the horse required an extended time to relax, and showed stiffness when turning to the right. According to the owner's observation, the problem with the back became apparent when the dressage saddle was changed to a jumping saddle.

Thermographic examination of the whole horse was performed at rest (Fig. 5.1) and after exercise (Fig 5.2). The thermograms indicated an increased circulation of the thoracic and lumbar vertebrae before and after exercise, with a significantly increased circulation in the thoracic vertebrae and back muscles after exercise. The examination also indicated increased circulation in the area of both sacroiliac joints when the thermograph was taken after 20 min of lunging, plus increased circulation on the left side of the croup (Fig. 5.2).

Muscle tension, as indicated by the thermographic examination, was confirmed by an equine physiotherapist. For the next 2 weeks, the horse was regularly lunged and had regular massage sessions. After 3 weeks, a further thermographic examination was performed, which indicated reduced circulation in the back, sacroiliac joints and the area of the left part of the croup. It was recommended that the horse be returned to work with a properly fitted saddle. After 1 month, the equine physiotherapist did not detect any tension or pain in the back and, according to the owner, the horse did not show any signs of stiffness while working under saddle.

CASE 2: MUSCLE TENSION OF THE CROUP   This horse was a 3-year-old Polish Halfbred gelding and was gradually being introduced to work under saddle. For the

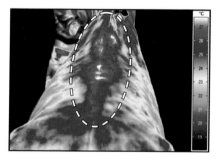

Fig. 5.1. Thermogram of the back and croup from the dorsal aspect before exercise. An increased body surface temperature of the thoracolumbar vertebrae and sacroiliac joints is indicated (dashed outline).

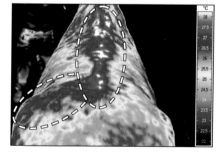

Fig. 5.2. Thermogram of the back and croup from the dorsal aspect after exercise. A increased body surface temperature of the thoracolumbar vertebrae, sacroiliac joints and left side of the croup is indicated (dashed outlines).

previous few weeks, the horse had not been sound on the right hindlimb. It was noted that the horse shortened his gait in the upper part of the limb, around the femur area. Veterinary examination of the stifle joint did not identify any signs of injury. The horse owner suspected a muscular problem, as the horse was not sound on soft ground.

Thermographic examination of the whole horse was performed at rest. The results of the examination indicated increased circulation on the right side of the flank (Fig. 5.3) compared with the left side (Fig. 5.4). The thermographic results were confirmed by an equine physiotherapist, who identified croup muscle tension around the flank. One week later, after regular massage sessions, the horse returned to work on the lunge without any signs of lameness of the right hindlimb.

CASE 3: FLEXOR TENDON OVERLOAD   This horse was a 4-year-old Thoroughbred stallion in intensive racing training. During training, the horse tended to reduce the load on the right forelimb. During a manual palpation examination, the horse had a painful reaction in the area of the third metacarpal bone.

Thermographic examination of the whole horse was performed at rest. The examination indicated increased circulation in the right limb in the area of the third metacarpal bone from the palmar aspect (Fig. 5.5). An ultrasonographic examination of the area identified by thermography confirmed a significant overload of the superficial digital flexor tendon. The horse was withdrawn from training for more than 2 months to allow recovery.

5.2 Manual Assessment of the Horse

Thermographic examination indicates areas with superficial temperature changes caused, in most cases, by muscle tension or healing processes. However, local temperature changes may not always indicate a tissue disorder or muscle regeneration. Conversely, lack of a local temperature change does not always indicate the absence of a problem. Therefore, after thermographic examination of the whole horse, a manual assessment (normally via palpation)

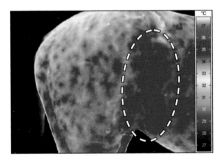

Fig. 5.3. Thermogram of the right side of the croup from the lateral aspect. An increased body surface temperature of the flank is indicated (dashed outline).

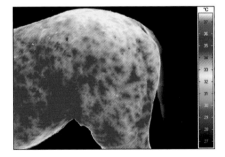

Fig. 5.4. Thermogram of the left side of the croup from the lateral aspect showing a normal body surface temperature of the flank.

of the areas of the body identified by the thermographic examination as potentially problematic should be performed in order to determine any discomfort, such as tension or pain in the soft tissues. Confirmation of the changes through palpation is a necessary complement for correct interpretation of the thermographic examination results.

Manual assessment allows the detection of any incorrect muscle function, including tissue tension and weakness. The tensioned tissue exhibits pain and stiffness on palpation, while weakened tissue has a lack of muscle strength and mass. Manual assessment of a horse is performed in five areas of the body: head, neck, forelimbs, back and hindlimbs.

In combination with thermography, manual assessment, largely through palpation to assess the skeletal and muscular system, should be performed as discussed in the following sections.

5.2.1   Head area

The skull of a horse is composed of two elements: the upper (immovable) part and the lower (movable) part (the mandible).

5.2.1.1   Skeletal system

The two parts of the skull are connected to each other through the temporomandibular joint, which acts like a hinge, allowing chewing movements, and gives the jaw the ability to move correctly from side to side, up and down, and backwards and forwards (Fig. 5.6). The temporomandibular joint mechanism does not operate independently but is connected to the rest of the body through a complicated set of structures – the stomatognathic system. This system consists of the parts of the head, neck and upper thorax, and comprises muscle, bone, ligaments and nerves. It controls biting, chewing and swallowing. It is made up of 27 bones, one of which is the mandible. The complex anatomical connections of the stomatognathic system mean that the proper function of the

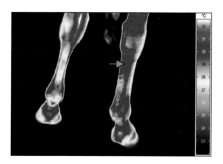

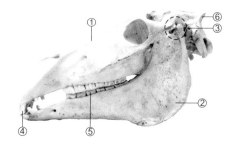

Fig. 5.5. Thermogram of the distal right and left forelimbs from the palmar aspect. Superficial digital flexor tendon overload of the right forelimb is indicated (green arrow).

Fig. 5.6. Skull from the left lateral aspect with the maxilla (1, upper jaw), mandible (2, lower jaw) and temporomandibular joint (3, dashed outline), incisors (4), molars (5) and poll area (6) indicated.

temporomandibular joint is dependent on the health of the back muscles and tendons, as well as the limb joints. This relationship also works the other way around: the proper function of the temporomandibular joint mechanism plays an important role in the function of the whole horse, including gait, balance and equilibrium.

The entire skull is connected to the spine at the poll area, which is responsible for flexion and extension movements, the so-called 'nodding' of the head.

5.2.1.2 Muscular system

The temporalis muscle is a small but very strong muscle with a thickness of about 2.5 cm. The function of this muscle is to close the mandible. The temporalis muscle works in conjunction with the major masseter muscle to bring the upper jaw and lower jaw together (Fig. 5.7). Contraction of the major masseter muscle lifts the lower jaw, pressing the canine and incisor teeth against each other, making the biting and chewing of food possible.

5.2.1.3 Indicators of a problem

Muscle and ligament tension of the temporomandibular joint is often indicated by misalignment of the upper and lower incisors (Fig. 5.8). This may be apparent from the wear of the teeth.

An overdeveloped temporalis muscle can indicate masseter muscle weakness due to dysfunction of the temporomandibular joint.

The poll area is an important site for insertion of the neck muscles as well as the nuchal ligament. Hypersensitivity of this area is often associated with strong neck muscle tension due to the constant effort required to lift the head up (in horses with high head carriage), or can be the result of problems in other body areas, such as muscle tension around the shoulders and back. Signs of poll hypersensitivity can include head shaking, crib biting and various behavioural problems.

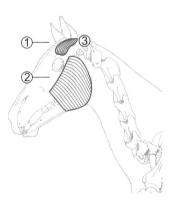

Fig. 5.7. Skull from the left lateral aspect with the temporalis muscle (1) and masseter muscle (2) indicated. Localization of muscle tension in the poll area is shown (3).

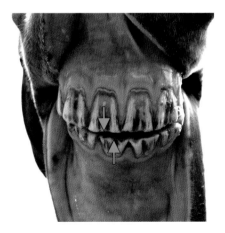

Fig. 5.8. Example of misalignment of the upper and lower incisors due to problems with the temporalis and/or masseter muscle.

5.2.1.4 Manual and visual assessment of the head
- Check for tension in the poll area by applying direct pressure (Fig 5.7).
- Check the alignment of the incisor teeth.
- Check for overdevelopment of the temporalis muscle.
- Assess for masseter muscle weakness.

5.2.2 Neck area

The neck consists of the seven cervical vertebrae, C1–C7.

5.2.2.1 Skeletal system
The first two cervical vertebrae (C1 and C2) are different from the other five. The first vertebra, C1 (the atlas) is connected to the poll area, forming the atlanto-occipital joint and enabling nodding of the head. Characteristically, the atlas lacks a vertebral body, which along with the second cervical vertebra, C2 (the axis), during the process of evolution has been modified into a tooth-like structure, creating the atlanto-axial joint. This joint gives the greatest mobility to neck movements and is responsible for head rotation and flexion. The other cervical vertebrae, C3–C7, have retained their vertebral body and are all similarly structured (Fig. 5.9). The upper surface of these vertebrae is uneven and rough, to enable insertion of the neck muscles and the nuchal ligament. The joints between cervical vertebrae C3–C7 allow lateral (side-to-side) flexion of the neck.

5.2.2.2 Muscular system
The brachiocephalicus muscle connects the head to the humerus. The main functions of this muscle are extension of the shoulder joint, moving the limb forward, and lateral neck movements.

   The main functions of the splenius muscle are moving the head up, straightening the neck, and flexion of the head and neck laterally (Fig. 5.10).

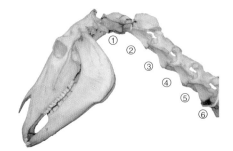

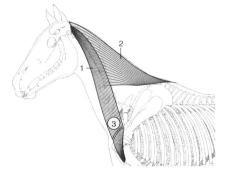

Fig. 5.9. Left side of the cervical vertebrae and skull from the lateral aspect showing the first cervical vertebra (C1, the atlas) (1), second cervical vertebra (C2, the axis) (2) and third (3), fourth (4), fifth (5) and sixth (6) cervical vertebrae (C3–C6). The seventh cervical vertebra (C7) is out of view.

Fig. 5.10. Left side of the neck from the lateral aspect showing the brachiocephalicus muscle (1) and splenius muscle (2). Localization of muscle tension in the base of the neck area is shown (3).

5.2.2.3 Indicators of a problem

Increased muscle tension in the atlanto-occipital joint area results in limitation of rotation and lateral flexion of the head. Muscle tension in this joint area can lead to disruption in the function of the atlanto-axial joint, resulting in tension of the splenius and brachiocephalicus muscles. This tension can spread to further neck areas (C3–C7), causing difficulties in lateral flexion of the neck, and affecting other back muscles, which may result in spasms of the back and croup area.

5.2.2.4 Manual and visual assessment of the neck

- Check for tension in the area of the base of the neck by applying direct pressure (Fig. 5.10).

5.2.3 Forelimb area

The main forelimb areas of concern are the shoulder and digit bones.

5.2.3.1 Skeletal system

The shoulder (or scapula) is a large triangular bone, with an ideal angle of slope of approximately 45°, and should be symmetrical for both shoulders (Fig. 5.11). This bone connects the forelimb to the spine via muscles, tendons, ligaments and fascia. This type of connection allows absorption of concussion and gives freedom of movement, as it enables both adduction and abduction of the limbs when the horse moves forwards and sideways.

The digit bones include the long pastern, short pastern and the coffin bone (Fig. 5.12). These bones absorb concussion. The long pastern is connected higher up the leg to the third metacarpal bone, forming the fetlock joint. The long pastern bone is also connected at the lower end to the short pastern bone below, forming the pastern joint. The short pastern bone is in turn connected to the coffin bone, forming the coffin joint. The short pastern is partially located in the hoof and is the first free bone, absorbing the concussion of the hoof on the ground. The joints of the digit bones have a very limited range of lateral and rotational movement, providing protection from subluxation.

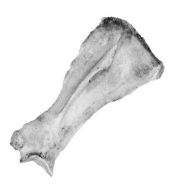

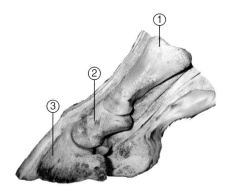

Fig. 5.12. Distal part of the forelimb from the lateral aspect showing the long pastern (1), short pastern (2) and coffin bone (3).

Fig. 5.11. Left scapula from the lateral aspect.

5.2.3.2 Muscular system

The muscular system of the shoulder area includes the muscles below the shoulder: the serratus ventralis cervicis and serratus ventralis thoracis muscles. The main functions of these muscles are suspension of the forelimb and shoulder movement backwards and forwards. The muscles above the shoulder have a similar function – the trapezius cervical and trapezius thoracic muscles draw the scapula backwards and forwards. The muscle in the elbow area, the triceps brachii, flexes the shoulder joint and extends the elbow joint, and at the same time provides elbow support (Fig. 5.13).

5.2.3.3 Indicators of a problem

A difference in the angle of the two shoulders or scapulae indicates asymmetrical development of the shoulder and back muscles. This results in uneven function of the forelimbs and a limited range of lateral flexion of the neck.

Uneven heels ('low heel/high heel' syndrome) can cause uneven absorption of concussion due to imbalance of limb function. The lower of the two heels will create obvious changes in the joint angles at the pastern, fetlock, elbow and shoulder joints when compared with the limb with the higher heel. The angles on the low-heeled limb will open (i.e. grow larger), and the limb will become more vertical than its counterpart throughout its length. The pastern and fetlock joints will be placed in greater extension, which is a possible cause of subluxation. The elbow angle will be more open. As the shoulder opens, the 'point' of the shoulder will be moved caudally so that its position is farther back than on the higher-heeled limb. The position of the scapula becomes altered so that it also becomes more vertical. This creates a bulging of the shoulder and overdevelopment of the associated muscles on the lower-heeled limb. This has a huge impact on muscle imbalance in the upper parts of the body and can cause changes in posture that result in loss of performance.

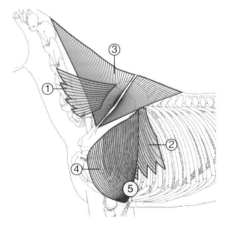

Fig. 5.13. Left side of the scapula from the lateral aspect showing the serratus ventralis cervicis muscle (1), serratus ventralis thoracis muscle (2), trapezius muscle (3) and triceps brachii muscle (4). Localization of muscle tension or weakness in the elbow joint area is indicated (5).

In addition, the lower heel is predisposed to tearing of the frog and can lead to incorrect functioning of the spine. The higher heel 'clubfoot' is more upright and absorbs more forceful concussion, as evidenced by a higher incidence of suspensory and check ligament injuries. This also correlates with the shortened stride as the shoulder takes proportionally more of the horse's weight.

5.2.3.4 Manual and visual assessment of the forelimb
- Check for muscle tissue tension or weakness in the area of the elbow joint by applying direct pressure (Fig. 5.13).
- Assess the angle of both shoulders.
- Check for low heel/high heel syndrome.

5.2.4 Back area

The main back area includes primarily the thoracic and lumbar vertebrae. Both parts of the spine are connected by strong muscles and ligaments.

5.2.4.1 Skeletal system
The thoracic spine consists of 18 vertebrae (Fig. 5.14), which are connected to each other via spinous processes. This region of the spine is characterized by limited mobility: only small vertical, horizontal and lateral movements are possible. The available flex between the joints is only 1–2°. Also characteristic for this spine region are very high spinous processes, the position of which depends on the neck position and head carriage. The withers (the highest part of the thoracic vertebrae) contain spinous processes that can reach a height of up to 25 cm. Therefore, this area is a good place for muscle, tendon and ligament attachment. The spinous processes in the second part of the thoracic vertebrae are smaller (Fig. 5.14). This section of the spine is subject to injuries such as inflammation of the spinous processes and back muscles, in many cases related to improper saddle fit.

The lumbar spine region consists of six vertebrae (Fig. 5.15). The spinous processes have a similar length to the spinous processes of the second part of the thoracic spine. However, the lumbar spine is characterized by long transverse processes, which act as insertion points for strong muscles, tendons and ligaments, characteristic of this region. The lumbar vertebrae form the least stable part of the spine due to a lack of bony connections and support. In contrast, the thoracic vertebrae are supported by a connection with the chest, and the sacral vertebrae are protected by a connection with the pelvis. The only

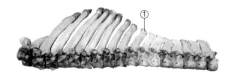

Fig. 5.14. Thoracic vertebrae from the lateral aspect with the spinous processes (1) indicated.

protection for internal organs lying below the lumbar vertebrae is that afforded by the muscles connected to the long transverse processes.

5.2.4.2 Muscular system

The function of the muscles surrounding the thoracic vertebrae is spine extension. They are also responsible for spine stabilization, and these muscles contribute to the transmission to the forelimbs of motion initiated in the hindlimbs.

One of the main back extensors is the longissimus dorsi muscle, which is the largest muscle in the back and plays an important role in the locomotor ability and performance of the horse. It extends bilaterally from the sacral to the cervical vertebrae. This muscle provides extension when bilaterally activated, and lateral flexion and axial rotation of the spine when unilaterally activated. It also stabilizes the back during movement of the horse. The iliocostalis dorsi muscle, located beneath the longissimus dorsi, is responsible for spine extension and lateral flexion of the thoracic region (Fig. 5.16).

The muscles of the cervical, thoracic and sacral vertebrae join together at the lumbar vertebrae. As a result, the main function of these muscles is transfer of the energy created by the hindlimbs to the forelimbs, which means they are the main driver of the body.

5.2.4.3 Indicators of a problem

The main dysfunction of the thoracic and lumbar region is spinous process subluxation or inflammation of the spinous processes (commonly referred to as kissing spine). This can be caused by: increased muscle tension around the neck, back and croup; poor conformation; sudden turns; slipping or falls; saddle-fit issues; improper hoof balance; injured limbs; or rider imbalance. Subluxation of the lumbar vertebrae causes muscle dysfunction in the hindlimbs, forelimbs, back and neck. Back muscle dysfunction in particular can have unrecognized ramifications, creating muscle imbalance and loss of performance, and can potentially lead to lameness.

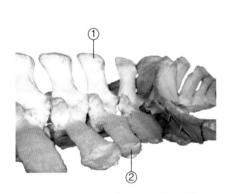

Fig. 5.15. Lumbar vertebrae from the lateral aspect with the spinous processes (1) and transverse processes (2) indicated.

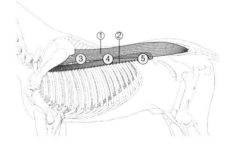

Fig. 5.16. Back from the lateral aspect showing the longissimus dorsi muscle (1) and iliocostalis dorsi muscle (2). Localization of muscle tension or muscle weakness in the withers area (3), caudal part of the thoracic vertebrae (4) and lumbar vertebrae (5) is indicated.

5.2.4.4   Manual and visual assessment of the back

- Check the thoracic and lumbar vertebrae spinous processes for subluxation.
- Check for muscle tension and swelling in the withers area by applying direct pressure (Fig. 5.16).
- Check for muscle tissue tension in the thoracic vertebrae by applying direct pressure (Fig. 5.16).
- Check for muscle tissue tension in the lumbar vertebrae by applying direct pressure (Fig. 5.16).

5.2.5   Hindlimb area

The main areas of concern in the hindlimb are the sacral vertebrae and pelvis.

5.2.5.1   Skeletal system

The last lumbar vertebra is connected to the sacrum, creating the lumbosacral joint. With the exception of the cervical and coccygeal vertebrae, this joint is the most flexible region of the spine, allowing the horse in motion to use its hindlimbs effectively and to round the back. This allows energy generated by the hindlimbs to be transferred effectively to the forelimbs. The flexion of this joint should be as great as possible to optimize athletic performance.

The sacrum is a triangular bone, which consists in most cases of five fused vertebrae. The first vertebra of the sacrum has a 'wing' (transverse process), which constitutes the link between the sacral bone and the pelvis. This is the sacroiliac joint, which is characterized by limited mobility. This joint is supported and stabilized by ventral, dorsal and sacroiliac ligaments and muscle insertions. These form strong connections between the hindlimb and spine, and transfer the energy generated by the hindlimbs to the forelimbs.

The pelvis consists of two pelvic bones, each of which is formed from three fused bones: the ilium, ischium and pubis. The ilium has palpable tuber coxae and tuber sacrale, which are the highest palpable points of the croup. At the level of the tuber sacrale, there is a link between the sacral bone and the pelvis. At the end of the ischium bone, there are palpable tuber ischii (Fig. 5.17). The fusion of the ilium, ischium and pubis forms the acetabulum, which in turn meets the head of the femur forming the hip joint. The hip is the largest and strongest joint in the body of the horse, characterized by high mobility.

5.2.5.2   Muscular system

The gluteus muscles covering the pelvis are strong muscles with a depth of up to 30 cm, and form the main propulsion force of the horse's body. The gluteus muscles include: the gluteus superficialis, responsible for flexion of the hip joint; the gluteus medialis, the largest in this muscle group, responsible for extension of the hip joint; and the gluteus profundus, responsible for abduction of the thigh (Figs 5.18 and 5.19).

The tensor fasciae latae muscle has its origin at the tuber coxae and is inserted at the patella, filling the space between the pelvis and femur. It is the main flexor of the hip joint (Fig. 5.18).

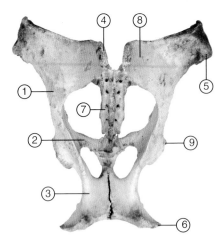

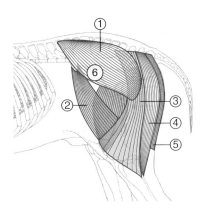

Fig. 5.17. Pelvis and sacrum from the dorsal aspect showing the ilium (1), pubis (2), ischium (3), tuber sacrale (4), tuber coxae (5), tuber ischia (6), sacral vertebrae (7), sacroiliac joint (8) and acetabulum (9).

Fig. 5.18. Croup from the lateral aspect showing the gluteus muscle group (1), tensor fasciae latae muscle (2), biceps femoris muscle (3), semitendinosus muscle (4) and semimembranosus muscle (5). Localization of gluteus muscles tension is indicated (6).

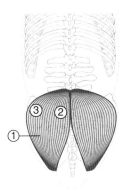

Fig. 5.19. Croup from the dorsal aspect showing the gluteus muscle group (1). Localization of muscle tension or weakness in the tuber sacrale (2) and tuber coxae (3) areas is indicated.

The hamstring group of muscles extend along the back of the hindlimb behind the hip joint, creating the muscle group responsible for extending the hip. The hamstring muscles consist of the biceps femoris, semitendinosus and semimembranosus muscles. These muscles play an important role in propelling the horse forward, extending and stabilizing the hip joint, flexing the stifle joint, and enabling abduction and adduction of the limb (Fig. 5.18).

5.2.5.3 Indicators of a problem

Strong tension of the gluteus muscles causes less efficient action of the hind-limbs or an uneven stride length. Tension of the ligaments and muscle in-sertions in the area of the tuber sacrale can indicate problems related to the function of the sacroiliac joints. Tension in the area of the tuber coxae in-dicates tension in the pelvic area. A difference in the level of the two tuber sacrales can indicate pelvic rotation, which affects the function of the liga-ments connecting the hip and sacral bone, causing an uneven load on the hip, stifle and tarsal joints.

5.2.5.4 Manual and visual assessment of the hindlimb

- Check for tension of the gluteus muscle group by applying direct pressure (Fig. 5.18).
- Check for tissue tension or weakness in the area of the tuber coxae and tuber sacrale by applying direct pressure (Fig. 5.19).
- Assess the level of the tuber sacrale.

5.3 Muscle Function

The horse functions as a coherent entity of muscle chains forming combined rows, which, when working together properly, enable balanced muscle work throughout the whole body. Disorders in muscle chain function are a conse-quence of injury (e.g. to bones, joints, and tendon structures around joints and ligaments), as well as compensation effects and long-term rehabilitation of the musculoskeletal and nervous systems.

5.3.1 Linked muscle function

The linked muscle function across the whole organism contributes to the rapid spread of efficient muscle activity, or inefficient activity in the case of abnor-malities. A good example of muscle chain activity connection is the frequent link between back and limb problems (and vice versa). The dysfunction of limb action can influence the appearance of disorders in the back. Initially, the horse may present with stiffness during work under saddle, have a lack of forward impulsion and need a long time to warm up. Later, the horse may shorten the stride and develop an uneven stride length, finally leading to injury of the mus-culoskeletal system. The more body areas that are affected by muscle tissue dis-orders, the more health problems appear, and it can then become more difficult to diagnose the true initial cause.

By way of illustration, the cases of five horses with diagnosed muscle ten-sion in various body areas arising from orthopaedic disorders are presented below. In all cases, after thermographic examination of the whole horse, manual assessment of the horse was carried out to confirm the thermographic results. This allowed the correct interpretation of the thermographic images in identifying musculoskeletal problems.

CASE 4: BACK SORENESS   This horse was a 14-year-old Polish Halfbred gelding in training for show jumping. The horse had the typical symptoms of back soreness: avoiding grooming, cold-backed when tacked up, stiffness of the body, poor hindlimb action and refusal to jump. Veterinary examination diagnosed spinous process inflammation in the withers area.

Thermographic examination of the whole horse at rest indicated increased circulation both in the withers area, where inflammation was diagnosed, and in the caudal part of the thoracic vertebrae, in which spinous process subluxation had occurred (Fig. 5.20). The examination also indicated increased blood circulation in the muscles in the croup area (gluteus muscles), especially on the right side (Figs 5.21 and 5.22). The increased muscle tension in the back area (because of spine inflammation) is likely in turn to have caused incorrect functioning of the gluteus muscles.

CASE 5: INFLAMMATION OF THE BRACHIOCEPHALICUS MUSCLE INSERTION   This horse was a 10-year-old Polish Halfbred mare. During exercise, the horse presented with tension throughout its whole body, especially in the poll area, and was very stiff on both reins but particularly on the right rein. On return of the horse after exercise, massage, together with ultrasound treatment, was being used on the poll area to try to regenerate muscle tissue and eliminate muscle tension.

Thermographic examination of the whole horse indicated increased circulation of the injured right side of the poll, which is the area of attachment of the brachiocephalicus muscle (Fig. 5.23). The thermographic images also indicated increased circulation of the right shoulder area, which is also an area of brachiocephalicus muscle attachment (Fig. 5.24).

The increased muscle tension in the poll area caused increased tension in the shoulder joint, thus shortening the stride of the right forelimb from the shoulder joint. This had the effect of incorrect distal limb action, causing increased circulation in the area of the third metacarpal bone (Fig. 5.25). Incorrect

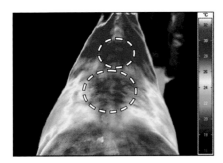

Fig. 5.20. Thermogram of the back from the dorsal aspect showing an increased body surface temperature in the withers area due to spinous process inflammation and a local increased body surface temperature in the caudal part of the thoracic vertebrae due to spinous process subluxation (dashed outlines).

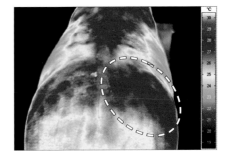

Fig. 5.21. Thermogram of the croup from the dorsal aspect. An increased body surface temperature of the gluteus muscles, especially in the right side of the croup, is indicated (dashed outline).

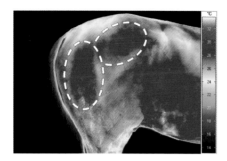

Fig. 5.22. Thermogram of the right side of the croup from the lateral aspect. An increased body surface temperature of the hip joint and tuber coxae area is indicated (dashed outlines).

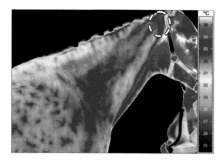

Fig. 5.23. Thermogram of the right side of the neck from the lateral aspect. An increased body surface temperature of the poll in the area of the brachio-cephalicus muscle origin is indicated (dashed outline).

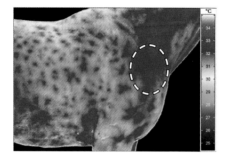

Fig. 5.24. Thermogram of the right side of the shoulder from the lateral aspect. An increased body surface temperature of the shoulder joint in the area of the brachiocephalicus muscle insertion is indicated (dashed outline).

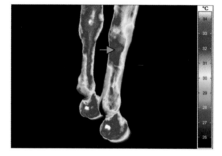

Fig. 5.25. Thermogram of the distal part of the right forelimb from the palmar aspect showing an increased body surface temperature of the third metacarpal bone (green arrow).

muscle function in the neck caused muscle tension around the back, resulting in spinous process subluxation in the thoracic and lumbar vertebrae (Fig. 5.26).

CASE 6: NAVICULAR BONE SYNDROME IN THE LEFT FORELIMB This horse was a 12-year-old Polish Halfbred gelding in dressage training. The horse was diagnosed with navicular bone syndrome in the left forelimb. After treatment, the horse returned to regular training, but during exercise, the horse was exhibiting muscle stiffness of the left forelimb, back and croup areas. It is likely that the pain from the navicular bone syndrome was forcing the horse to land on the toe instead of the heel, which resulted in shortening of the stride and uneven absorption of concussion, in turn causing incorrect function of muscles in the shoulder area.

After thermographic examination of the whole horse, increased circulation of the left hoof sole in the area of the toe was detected, confirming that the horse was still working incorrectly by landing on the toe (Fig. 5.27). The dysfunction of the hoof caused incorrect function of the soft tissue in the left limb in the area of the third metacarpal bone and shoulder muscles (Figs 5.28 and 5.29). Imbalance in forelimb function contributed to strong muscle tension in the back area, causing spinous process subluxation in the thoracic vertebrae, as well as muscle tension in the croup area, which was confirmed by the thermographic examination (Figs 5.30 and 5.31).

CASE 7: SUPERFICIAL DIGITAL FLEXOR TENDON INJURY IN THE RIGHT FORELIMB   This horse was an 18-year-old Polish Halfbred mare in light training for pleasure riding. After the initial injury, the horse was rested for 5 months. After tendon recovery, the horse returned to regular but light work. Within a few weeks, however, the mare was unsound again on the right forelimb. Veterinary examination did not indicate any injury or any other possible reason for the lameness.

After thermographic examination of the whole horse, increased circulation in the area of the third metacarpal bone of the right forelimb was indicated (Fig. 5.32),

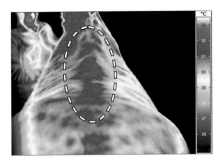

Fig. 5.26. Thermogram of the back from the dorsal aspect showing an increased body surface temperature of the thoracolumbar vertebrae due to spinous process subluxation (dashed outline).

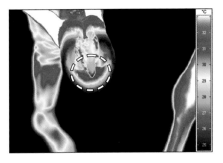

Fig. 5.27. Thermogram of the left front hoof from the solar aspect. An increased body surface temperature of the toe is indicated (dashed outline).

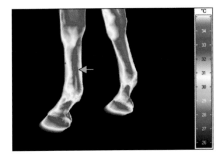

Fig. 5.28. Thermogram of the distal part of the left and right forelimbs from the lateral and medial aspects, respectively. An increased body surface temperature of left third metacarpal bone is indicated (green arrow).

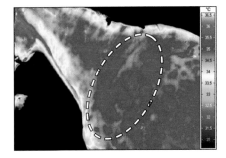

Fig 5.29. Thermogram of the left side of the shoulder from the lateral aspect. An increased body surface temperature of the shoulder muscles in the area of the scapula is indicated (dashed outline).

in the area of the previous tendon injury. In addition, the examination detected increased circulation in the atlanto-axial joint and in the withers area of the thoracic vertebrae (Figs 5.33 and 5.34). It was evident that the incorrect functioning of the right forelimb had caused muscle function imbalance in the neck and back. Ultrasonographic examination carried out by a veterinarian confirmed a repeat injury of the superficial digital flexor tendon in the exact area indicated by the thermographic examination. The repeated injury was probably caused by incomplete healing of the injured tendon.

CASE 8: NAVICULAR SYNDROME IN THE RIGHT FORELIMB   This horse was a 7-year-old Polish Halfbred gelding with a previous navicular syndrome diagnosis (2 years ago). During treatment, the horse was diagnosed with spinous process inflammation of the thoracic vertebrae. Once treatment of the navicular syndrome was successfully completed, the horse had returned to regular training. However, he presented with shortened strides and stiffness of the right forelimb, especially

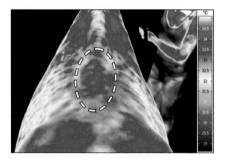

Fig. 5.30. Thermogram of the back from the dorsal aspect. An increased body surface temperature of the thoracic vertebrae due to spinous process subluxation is indicated (dashed outline).

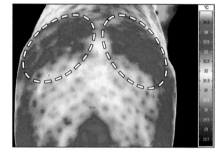

Fig. 5.31. Thermogram of the croup from the dorsal aspect. An increased body surface temperature of the croup muscles is indicated (dashed outline).

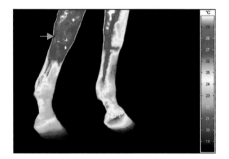

Fig. 5.32. Thermogram of the distal part of the right and left forelimbs from the lateral and medial aspects, respectively. An increased body surface temperature of right third metacarpal bone is indicated (green arrow).

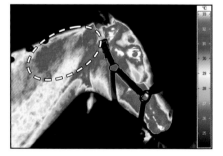

Fig. 5.33. Thermogram of the right side of neck and head from the lateral aspect. An increased body surface temperature in the area of the atlanto-axial joint is indicated (dashed outline).

when taking turns to the left, and had a lack of forward impulsion. On soft ground, the horse was not sound on the right forelimb, which initially indicated a soft tissue problem. According to the owner's observations, the horse was sound on the right forelimb during exercise after a long warm-up. At the end of exercise, the horse was soft and flexible throughout his body. Veterinary examination did not indicate any changes in the suspect right hoof. Examination of the back and neck areas also did not indicate any injuries.

Thermographic examination of the whole horse did not indicate any signs of injury of the right forelimb. However, increased circulation was indicated on the right side of the neck, above the cervical vertebrae (Fig. 5.35). This was probably caused by unbalanced function of the neck muscles due to the horse landing on the right toe instead of the heel because of the navicular pain. This had resulted in overdevelopment of the muscles on the right side of the neck. The back injury, which occurred during treatment for navicular syndrome, was probably a consequence of uneven forelimb stride length, resulting in loss of balance and incorrect function of the spine. After regular daily massage treatments, the horse gradually returned to work.

5.3.2 Antagonistic muscle function

Antagonistic muscles exemplify the co-ordination of the muscular system and consist of two muscle groups working in opposition. In any initiated motion, one muscle is responsible for flexion and the other for extension movements. This co-ordination results in balanced, precise and controlled movement. An example of antagonistic muscles is the flexor and extensor muscles of the back. These groups, working in opposite directions, create separate muscle chains.

The back extensor muscles include the muscles located along the spine, the main function of which is both extension and stabilization of the spine. They extend from the sacral and hip bones along the thoracic and lumbar vertebrae,

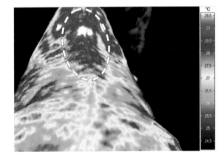

Fig. 5.34. Thermogram of the back from the dorsal aspect. An increased body surface temperature of the thoracic vertebrae, also in the withers area, is indicated (dashed outline).

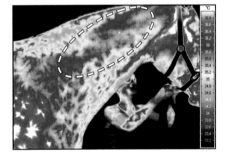

Fig. 5.35. Thermogram of the right side of the neck from the lateral aspect. An increased body surface temperature of the neck muscles is indicated (dashed outline).

and connect to the cervical vertebrae (Fig. 5.36). These paired muscle blocks are situated on both sides of the body, and comprise:

- the longissimus dorsi muscle, providing extension when bilaterally active, and lateral flexion and axial rotation to the spine when unilaterally active; it also stabilizes the back during movement of the horse;
- the iliocostalis dorsi muscle, responsible for extension and lateral flexion of the spine; and
- the spinalis dorsi muscle, responsible for extension of the thoracic and lumbar vertebrae.

The muscle chain of back extensors is responsible for gymnastic movements and support of the spine. These muscles transmit the energy of motion, initiated in the hindlimbs, to the forelimbs. They also contribute to forward movement, especially during canter and jumping.

The back flexor muscles include muscles located under the chest from the sternum to the ilium area. They are responsible for flexion and support of the spine (Fig. 5.36). These comprise:

- the rectus abdominis muscle, which is responsible for flexion and support of the spine;
- the obliquus internus abdominis and obliquus externus abdominis muscles, which flex the spine, support the chest and compress the abdominal viscera; and
- the transversus abdominis muscle, which flexes the spine and supports respiration.

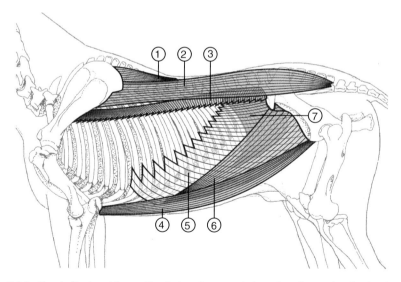

Fig. 5.36. The left chest from the lateral aspect showing the spinalis dorsi muscle (1), longissimus dorsi muscle (2), iliocostalis dorsi muscle (3), rectus abdominis muscle (4), obliquus externus abdominis muscle (5), obliquus internus abdominis muscle (6) and transversus abdominis muscle (7).

The muscle chain of back flexors plays an important role in forming and supporting the spine's shape and position. These muscles are also important in movements necessary to carry the rider and movements to support respiration. The back flexors and extensors form joint chains of antagonistic muscles, which, when interacting properly, enable the horse to balance correctly. Strong tension of the extensors of the back muscles can occur frequently during exercise due to incorrect function of the musculoskeletal system. The appearance of increased tension in one of the extensor muscles causes a knock-on dysfunction of the other muscles in the chain. Constant extensor muscle tension has a negative impact on the function of their antagonistic muscles – the abdominal flexors – causing dysfunction, leading to abnormal movement. This is because of a simple mechanism: the contraction of one muscle group causes the automatic simultaneous relaxation of their antagonistic muscles. When a given group of muscles remains in chronic tension for a prolonged period of time (months or years), their antagonists, in accordance with this principle, are in automatic relaxation and gradually weaken over time. Their activity therefore decreases in proportion to the overactivity of the antagonistic muscles.

By way of illustration, the cases of two horses with dysfunction of the antagonistic flexors and extensors of the back are presented below. During training both horses presented with stiffness and had problems in returning to flexibility. Manual assessment of both horses demonstrated soreness and strong tension of the back muscles in the area of the thoracic vertebrae.

CASES 9 AND 10: DYSFUNCTION OF THE ANTAGONISTIC FLEXORS AND EXTENSORS OF THE BACK   Case 9 was an 8-year-old Polish Halfbred gelding in training for show jumping (Figs 5.37–5.39). Case 10 was a 12-year-old Polish Halfbred gelding in training for dressage and for leisure riding (Figs 5.40–5.42).

In both cases, incorrect muscle function in the back area, accompanied by incorrect function of their antagonistic muscles in the abdomen area, was indicated by thermographic examination. Soreness and tension of the back muscles in

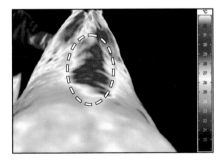

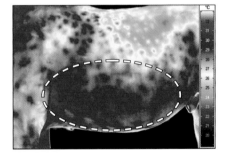

Fig. 5.37. Thermogram of the back from the dorsal aspect. An increased body surface temperature of the thoracic vertebrae on the horse's right hand side due to back muscle tension is indicated (dashed outline).

Fig. 5.38. Thermogram of the left side of the chest from the lateral aspect. An increased body surface temperature of the abdominal muscles is indicated (dashed outline).

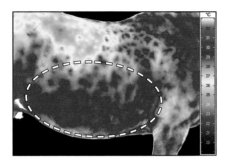

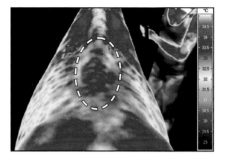

Fig. 5.39. Thermogram of the right side of the chest from the lateral aspect. An increased body surface temperature of the abdominal muscles is indicated (dashed outline).

Fig. 5.40. Thermogram of the back from the dorsal aspect. An increased body surface temperature of the thoracic vertebrae due to back muscle tension is indicated (dashed outline).

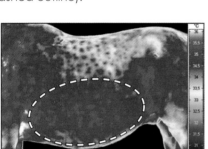

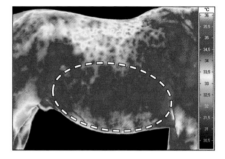

Fig. 5.41. Thermogram of the left side of the chest from the lateral aspect. An increased body surface temperature of the abdominal muscles is indicated (dashed outline).

Fig. 5.42. Thermogram of the right side of the chest from the lateral aspect. An increased body surface temperature of the abdominal muscles is indicated (dashed outline).

the thoracic vertebrae prevented proper functioning of the abdominal muscles, reducing work efficiency.

5.3.3 Diagonal limb muscle function

Dysfunction of diagonal limb muscles is often apparent in limb injuries. Tension and muscle weakness in the injured limb can disturb the function of muscles or joints in the diagonal limb. This causes improper balance of the diagonal limb and also the spine, as it connects the forelimbs and hindlimbs and attempts to compensate to restore biomechanical balance. Motion initiated by a hindlimb involves muscles, tendons and ligaments along the spine, transferring muscle action to the diagonal forelimb (Fig. 5.43) (Denoix, 1999; Faber et al., 2001). There is a similar association between the body surface temperature of the forelimbs, hindlimbs and spine (Soroko et al., 2015).

Work at trot and canter demonstrates the diagonal association of the limbs. Trot is a two-beat gait involving diagonal pairs of legs: right hindlimb–left forelimb and left hindlimb–right forelimb. Canter is a three-beat gait and when on the right lead, the horse loads the left hindlimb in the first stage, two diagonal limbs in the second stage (the right hindlimb and left forelimb) and finally the right forelimb in the last stage. Therefore, limb injury can contribute to functional disorders of the diagonal limb, resulting in poor gait of both limbs. Initially, the horse typically presents with stiffness during exercise and needs a prolonged time to warm up. Later, the horse is stiff throughout the body, has difficulties with lateral movements, lacks forward impulsion and has poor hindlimb engagement.

By way of illustration, the cases of three horses with diagonal limb problems are presented below. The thermographic examination results were confirmed by manual assessment of the horse or by routine veterinary examination.

CASE 11: LACK OF POLL FLEXION AND DECREASED LATERAL NECK FLEXION   This horse was a 14-year-old Thoroughbred gelding in light training for leisure riding. The horse had not been sound on the left forelimb for a prolonged period of time. Moreover the horse was tripping on both forelimbs during work under saddle, as well as during lunging. The horse presented with a lack of poll flexion and a lack of lateral neck flexion to the right.

Thermographic examination of the whole horse indicated an increased surface body temperature of the left forelimb in the area of the third metacarpal bone and fetlock joint (Fig. 5.44). The diagonal limb of the left forelimb, the right hindlimb, had an increased body surface temperature in the hip joint area

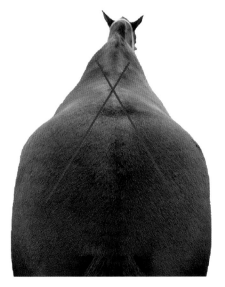

Fig. 5.43. Diagram of the back and croup from the dorsal aspect. The arrows link the antagonistic (diagonal) limbs: right forelimb and left hindlimb, and left forelimb and right hindlimb.

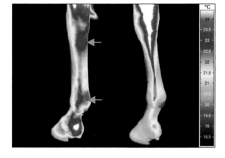

Fig. 5.44. Thermogram of the distal left and right forelimbs from the palmar aspect. An increased body surface temperature of the left third metacarpal bone (green arrow) and fetlock joint (blue arrow) of the left forelimb is indicated.

(Fig. 5.45). This problem of the diagonal limbs caused an increased body surface temperature of the thoracic and lumbar vertebrae (Fig. 5.46).

CASE 12: INFLAMMATION OF THE SUSPENSORY LIGAMENT   This horse was a 10-year-old Polish Halfbred gelding diagnosed with calcification of the proximal sesamoids and inflammation of the suspensory ligament in the right forelimb. Shortly after completing treatment of the right forelimb, the horse developed severe pain in the thoracic vertebrae, especially in the withers area. The horse was stiff throughout his body during exercise and had poor engagement of the hindlimbs. According to the observations of the owner, the horse worked more efficiently after warming up.

Thermographic examination of the whole horse indicated an increased body surface temperature of the fetlock joint of the right forelimb (Fig. 5.47). Increased circulation in the stifle and fetlock joint of the diagonal hindlimb was also indicated (Figs 5.48 and 5.49). Thermographic examination of the back indicated increased circulation of the thoracic and lumbar vertebrae

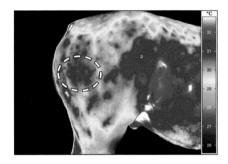

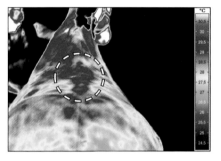

Fig. 5.45. Thermogram of the right side of the croup from the lateral aspect. An increased body surface temperature of the hip joint is indicated (dashed outline).

Fig. 5.46. Thermogram of the back and croup from the dorsal aspect. An increased body surface temperature of the thoracolumbar vertebrae is indicated (dashed outline).

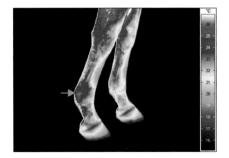

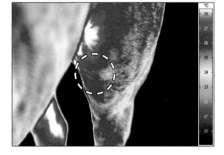

Fig. 5.47. Thermogram of the distal right and left forelimbs from the lateral and medial aspects, respectively. An increased body surface temperature of the right fetlock joint is indicated (green arrow).

Fig. 5.48. Thermogram of the left stifle joint from the dorsal aspect. An increased body surface temperature of the stifle joint is indicated (dashed outline).

(Fig. 5.50), as well as increased vascularization in the area of the left sacro-iliac joint (Fig. 5.51).

CASE 13: PELVIC ROTATION   This horse was a 5-year-old Polish Halfbred gelding diagnosed with pelvic rotation and treated by an equine chiropractor for pelvis relocation.

When the horse returned to regular light training after treatment, he had a shortened stride on the right hindlimb. Thermographic examination of the whole horse indicated an increased body surface temperature of the right croup area (Figs 5.52 and 5.53). Consequently, the limb diagonal to this area, the left forelimb, had an increased body surface temperature from the carpal joint to the hoof (Fig 5.54). The spine, as the connecting element of the two limbs, had an increased body surface temperature in the thoracic vertebrae (Fig. 5.55).

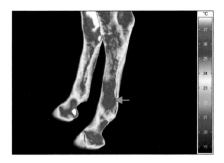

Fig. 5.49. Thermogram of the distal left and right forelimbs from the lateral and medial aspects, respectively. An increased body surface temperature of the left fetlock joint is indicated (blue arrow).

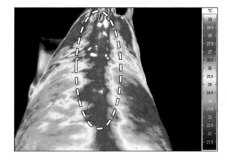

Fig. 5.50. Thermogram of the back from the dorsal aspect. An increased body surface temperature of the thoracolumbar vertebrae is indicated (dashed outline).

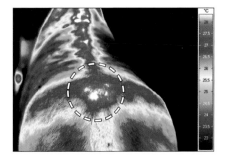

Fig. 5.51. Thermogram of the croup from the dorsal aspect. An increased body surface temperature of the left sacroiliac joint is indicated (dashed outline).

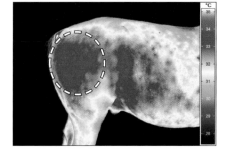

Fig. 5.52. Thermogram of the right side of the croup from the lateral aspect. An increased body surface temperature of the croup area is indicated (dashed outline).

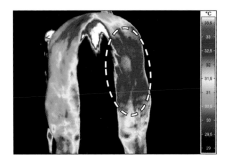

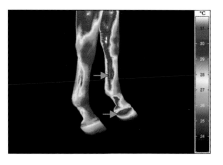

Fig. 5.53. Thermogram of the croup from the caudal aspect. An increased body surface temperature of the right side of the croup is indicated (dashed outline).

Fig. 5.54. Thermogram of the distal left and right forelimbs from the lateral and medial aspects, respectively. An increased body surface temperature of the left forelimb in the area between carpal joint and hoof is indicated (blue arrows).

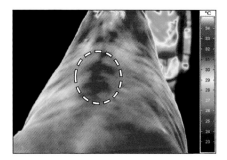

Fig. 5.55. Thermogram of the back from the dorsal aspect. An increased body surface temperature of the thoracic vertebrae is indicated (dashed outline).

5.4   Dysfunction of the Musculoskeletal System: Summary

Thermographic examination of the whole horse allows determination of the physiological nature of the tissue problems across a horse, as well as indicating specific body areas with incorrect function of the musculoskeletal system.

The cases presented above confirmed that incorrect tissue function in one body area caused dysfunction in another area. It is important to remember that correct diagnosis is dependent on complete knowledge of horse anatomy, with a special emphasis on the musculoskeletal system and biomechanics. Thermography enables quick, non-invasive and safe identification of body areas that have undergone physiological change or injury requiring further diagnosis or treatment. Regular application of thermographic examination helps to locate the body areas potentially susceptible to injury and, in the case of an injury, to monitor treatment progress. It helps the equine physiotherapist to determine the body areas requiring attention to aid quick and efficient recovery of the horse, and return it to its full athletic performance. In veterinary practice, thermography is a supplementary diagnostic tool, and can help to confirm the results of routine veterinary examinations.

It should be noted that thermography is a good preventative as well as diagnostic tool with a real role to play in sport and racehorse training centres and veterinary practice. It can be used as a supplementary tool to routine radiographic and ultrasonographic examinations, allowing the site of an injury to be determined, whereas radiographic and ultrasonographic examination can be used to determine the nature of the injury.

6 Recommendations for Thermography Application

In summary, the use of thermography may prove particularly useful for the following:

- Diagnosis of limb injuries: abscesses, laminitis, navicular bone syndrome, tendon and ligament inflammation, and stifle, carpal and tarsal joint inflammation.
- Diagnosis of back injuries: spinous process inflammation, supraspinal and interspinal ligament inflammation and intervertebral inflammation of the thoracolumbar vertebrae, back muscle inflammation and sacroiliac joint injury.
- Diagnosis of neurological disease.
- Detection of subclinical inflammation, allowing protection of the horse from serious injury or extended healing times.
- Monitoring of treatment, in particular anti-inflammatory drug effectiveness, informing managers and thus ensuring adequate time is allowed for full recovery.
- Monitoring the impact of training, in particular the impact of exercise overload, horse adaptation to training overload and evaluation of proper muscle balance.
- Monitoring of skin wounds on the limbs under dressings/casts.
- Assessing internal body temperature, indicated by the surface temperature at the corner of the eye.
- Detection of illegal topical chemical use, recommended by the International Equestrian Federation (FEI), which uses thermography for easier detection of artificially induced temperature changes, particularly in jumping horses.
- Assessing the correctness of saddle fitting.
- Assessing hoof function, both unshod and shod, in particular the impact on blood circulation in the distal limbs.

© M. Soroko and M.C.G. Davies Morel 2016. *Equine Thermography in Practice* (M. Soroko and M.C.G. Davies Morel)

References

American Academy of Thermology (2013) *Veterinary Guidelines for Infrared Thermography.* <http://www.aathermology.org/organization/guidelines/veterinary-guidelines-for-infrared-thermography> (accessed 15 December 2014).

Arruda, T.Z., Brass, K.E. and de la Corte, F.D. (2011) Thermographic assessment of saddles used on jumping horses. *Journal of Equine Veterinary Science* 31, 625–629.

Bathe, P.A. (2007) Thermography. In: Floyd, A. and Mansmann, R. (eds) *Equine Podiatry*. Saunders (an imprint of Elsevier), St Louis, Missouri, pp. 167–170.

Bowman, K.F., Purohit, R.C., Ganjam, V.K., Pechman, R.D. and Vaughan, J.T. (1983) Thermographic evaluation in corticosteroid efficacy in amphotericin B-induced arthritis in ponies. *American Journal of Veterinary Research* 44, 51–56.

Cena, K. (1974) Radiative heat loss from animal and man. In: Monteih J.L. and Mount, L.E (eds) *Heat Loss From Animals and Man*. Butterworths, London, UK, pp. 34–57.

Cena, K. and Clark, J.A. (1973) Thermal radiation from animal coat: coat structure and measurement of radiative temperature. *Physics in Medicine and Biology* 18, 432–443.

Cena, K. and Monteith, J.L. (1975) Transfer processes in animal coats. I. Radiative transfer. *Proceedings of the Royal Society B: Biological Sciences* 188, 377–393.

Clark, J.A. and Cena, K. (1977) The potential of infra-red thermography in veterinary diagnosis. *Veterinary Record* 100, 402–404.

Davy, J.R. (1977) Medical application of thermography. *Physics in Technology* 3, 54–61.

De Cocq, P., van Weeren, P.R. and Back, W. (2004) Effects of girth, saddle and weight on movements of the horse. *Equine Veterinary Journal* 36, 758–763.

Delahanty, D.D. and Georgi, J.R. (1965) Thermography in equine medicine. *Journal of the American Veterinary Medical Association* 147, 235–238.

Denoix, J.M. (1999) Spinal biomechanics and functional anatomy. *Veterinary Clinics of North America: Equine Practice* 15, 27–60.

Draper, J.W. and Boag, J.W. (1971a) The calculation of skin temperature distributions in thermography. *Physics in Medicine and Biology* 16, 201–211.

Draper, J.W. and Boag, J.W. (1971b) Skin temperature distributions over veins and tumours. *Physics in Medicine and Biology* 16, 645–654.

Eddy, A.L., van Hoogmoed, L.M. and Snyder, J.R. (2001) The role of thermography in the management of equine lameness. *Veterinary Journal* 162, 172–181.

Estberg, L., Gardner, I.A., Stover, S.M., Johnson, B.J., Case, J.T. and Ardans, A. (1995) Cumulative racing – seed distance cluster as a risk factor for fatal musculoskeletal injury in thoroughbred racehorses in California. *Preventive Veterinary Medicine* 24, 253–263.

Evans, G.P., Behiri, J.C., Vaughan, L.C., Vaughan, L.C. and Bonfield, W. (1992) The response of equine cortical bone to loading at strain rates experienced in vivo by the galloping horse. *Equine Veterinary Journal* 24, 125–128.

Faber, M., Johnston, C., Schamhardt, H.C., van Weeren, P.R., Roepstorff, L. and Barneveld, A. (2001) Three-dimensional kinematics of the equine spine during canter. *Equine Veterinary Journal Supplement* 33, 145–149.

Fleischmann, T., Siewert, C., Staszyk, C., Schulze, M., Stadler, P. and Seifert, H. (2009) Thermal imaging as an aid to the diagnosis of pain in horses – first results. In: *World Congress on Medical Physics and Biomedical Engineering, 7–12 September, 2009, Munich, Germany.* IFMBE Proceedings 25/2, 277–280.

Flores, S.C. (1978) Beruhrungslose temperaturmessung an der haut oberfläche beim pferd. klinik fúe pferde der tierärztlichen hochschule. Veterinary Medicine Dissertation.

Fonseca, B.P.A., Alves, A.L.G., Nicoletti, J.L.M., Thomassian, A., Hussini, C.A. and Mikaik, S. (2006) Thermography and ultrasonography in back pain diagnosis of equine athletes. *Journal of Equine Veterinary Science* 26, 507–516.

Ghafir, Y., Art, T. and Lekeus, P. (1996) Thermography facial patterns following an α2-adrenergic agonist injection on two horses suffering from Horner's syndrome. *Equine Veterinary Journal* 8, 192–195.

Harman, J.C. (1999) Tack and saddle fit. In: Turner, S. and Haussler, K.K. (eds) *Veterinary Clinics of North America. Equine Practice. Back Problems.* Saunders, Philadelphia, Pennsylvania, pp. 247–261.

Haussler, K.K, Stover, S.M. and Willits, N.H. (1999) Pathology of the lumbosacral spine and pelvis in thoroughbred racehorses. *American Journal of Veterinary Research* 60, 143–153.

Haussler, K.K., Bertram, J.E.A., Gellman, K. and Hermanson, J.W. (2001) Segmental *in vivo* vertebral kinematics at the walk, trot and canter: a preliminary study. *Equine Veterinary Journal Supplement* 33, 160–164.

Head, J. and Dyson, S. (2001) Taking the temperature of equine thermography. *Veterinary Journal* 162, 166–167.

International Equestrian Federation (2015) *Limb Sensitivity in Equestrian Competition.* <http://www.fei.org/fei/your-role/veterinarians/limb-sensitivity> (accessed 4 June 2015).

Ivanov, K.P. (2006) The development of the concepts of homeothermy and thermoregulation. *Journal of Thermal Biology* 31, 24–29.

Jeffcott, L.B., Dalin, G., Ekman, S. and Olsson, S.E. (1985) Sacroiliac lesions as a cause of chronic poor performance in competitive horses. *Equine Veterinary Journal* 17, 111–118.

Jodkowska, E. (2005) Body surface temperature as a criterion of the horse predisposition to effort. *Zeszyty Naukowe Akademii Rolniczej we Wrocławiu* 511, 7–114 (in Polish with English abstract).

Jodkowska, E. and Dudek, K. (2000) [Study on symmetry of body surface temperature of race horses]. *Przegląd Naukowej Literatury Zootechnicznej* 50, 307–319 (in Polish).

Johnson, S.R., Rao, S., Hussey, S.B., Morley, P.S. and Traub-Dargatz, J.L. (2011) Thermographic eye temperature as an index to body temperature in ponies. *Journal of Equine Veterinary Science* 31, 63–66.

Kastberger, G. and Stachl, R. (2003) Infrared imaging technology and biological applications. *Behavior Research Methods, Instruments, & Computers* 35, 429–439.

Katayama, Y., Ishida, N., Kaneko, M., Yamaoka, S. and Oikawa, M. (2001) The influence of exercise intensity on bucked shin complex in horses. *Journal of Equine Science* 12, 139–143.

Kold, S.E. and Chappell, K.A. (1998) Use of computerized thermographic image analysis (CTIA) in equine orthopedics: review and presentation of clinical cases. *Equine Veterinary Education* 10, 198–204.

Latif, S.N., von Peinen, K., Wiestner, T., Bitschnau, C., Renk, B. and Weishaupt, M.A. (2010) Saddle pressure patterns of three different training saddles (normal tree, flexible tree, treeless) in Thoroughbred racehorses at trot and gallop. *Equine Veterinary Journal* 42, 630–636.

Lawson, R.N. (1956) Implications of surface temperatures in the diagnosis of breast cancer. *Canadian Medical Association Journal* 75, 309–310.

Levet, T., Martens, A., Devisschear, L., Duchateur, L., Bogaert, L. and Vlamink, L. (2009). Distal limb cast sores in horses: risk factors and early detection using thermography. *Equine Veterinary Journal* 41, 18–23.

Magnusson, L.E. (1985) Studies on the conformation and related traits of Standardbred trotters in Sweden. IV. Relationship between conformation and soundness of 4-year-old Standardbred trotters. Master's thesis, Swedish University of Agricultural Sciences, Skara, Sweden.

McGreevy, P., Warren-Smith, A. and Guisard, Y. (2012) The effect of double bridles and jaw-clamping crank nosebands on temperature of eyes and facial skin of horses. *Journal of Veterinary Behavior* 7, 142–148.

Mogg, K.C. and Pollitt, C.C. (1992) Hoof and distal limb surface temperature in the normal pony under constant and changing ambient temperature. *Equine Veterinary Journal* 24, 134–139.

Nelson, H.A. and Osheim, D.L. (1975) *Soring in Tennessee Walking Horses: Detection by Thermography*. US Department of Agriculture, Animal and Plant Health Inspection Service, Veterinary Services Laboratories Ames, Iowa.

Palmer, S.E. (1981) Use of portable infrared thermometer as a means of measuring limb surface temperature in the horse. *American Journal of Veterinary Research* 42, 105–108.

Palmer, S.E. (1983) Effect of ambient temperature upon the surface temperature of the equine limb. *American Journal of Veterinary Research* 44, 1098–1101.

Peham, C., Kotschwar, A.B., Borkenhagen, B., Kuhnke, S., Molsner, J. and Baltacis, A. (2010) A comparison of forces acting on the horse's back and the stability of the rider's seat in different positions at the trot. *Veterinary Journal* 184, 56–59.

Peloso, J.G., Mundy, G.D. and Cohen, N.D. (1994) Prevalence of, and factors associated with, musculoskeletal racing injuries of Thoroughbreds. *Journal of the American Medical Association* 204, 620–626.

Purohit, R.C. (2008) Use of thermography in veterinary medicine. In: Cohen, J.M. and Lee, M. (eds) *Thermography in Rehabilitation Medicine*. Impress Publication, Wilsonville, Oregon, pp. 135–147.

Purohit, R.C. (2009) Standards for thermal imaging in veterinary medicine. In: *Proceedings of the 11th European Congress of Thermology*, 17–20 September, Mannheim, Germany, p. 99.

Purohit, R.C. and McCoy, M.D. (1980) Thermography in the diagnosis of inflammatory process in the horse. *American Journal of Veterinary Research* 41, 1167–1174.

Purohit, R.C., McCoy, M.D. and Bergfeld, W.A. (1980) Thermographic diagnosis of Horner's syndrome in the horse. *American Journal of Veterinary Research* 41, 1180–1182.

Purohit, R.C., Pascoe, D.D., DeFranco, B. and Schumacher, J. (2004) Thermographic evaluation of the neurovascular System of the equine. *Thermology International* 14, 89–92.

Ring, F.J. (1990) Quantitative thermal imaging. *Clinical Physics and Physiological Measurement* 11, 87–97.

Ring, F.J. (2007) The historical development of temperature measurement in medicine. *Infrared Physics and Technology* 49, 297–301.

Ring, F.J. and Ammer, K. (2012) Infrared thermal imaging in medicine. *Physiological Measurement* 33, R33–R46.

Rogalski, A. (2011) Recent progress in infrared detector technologies. *Infrared Physics and Technology* 54, 136–154.

Scott, M. and Swenson, L.A. (2009) Evaluating the benefits of equine massage therapy: a review of the evidence and current practices. *Journal of Equine Veterinary Science* 29, 687–697.

Simon, E.L., Gaughan, E.M., Epp, T. and Spire, M. (2006) Influence of exercise on thermographic-ally determined surface temperatures of thoracic and pelvic limbs in horses. *Journal of the American Veterinary Medicine Association* 229, 1940–1944.

Smith, W.M. (1964) Application of thermography in veterinary medicine. *Annals of the New York Academy of Sciences* 121, 248–254.

Soroko, M. (2011a) [Thermographic diagnosis of sport horses' limbs]. *Inżynieria Biomedyczna* 17, 104–109 (in Polish).

Soroko, M. (2011b) [Analysis of superficial temperature distribution of lower part of the limbs in young racehorses]. *Pomiary, Automatyka, Kontrola* 57, 1157–1160 (in Polish).

Soroko, M., Jodkowska, E. and Zabłocka, M. (2012) The use of thermography to evaluate back mus-culoskeletal responses of young racehorses to training. *Thermology International* 22, 152–156.

Soroko, M., Henklewski, R., Filipowski, H. and Jodkowska, E. (2013) The effectiveness of thermo-graphic analysis in equine orthopedics. *Journal of Equine Veterinary Science* 33, 760–762.

Soroko, M., Dudek, K., Howell, K., Jodkowska, E. and Henklewski, R. (2014) Thermographic evaluation of racehorse performance. *Journal of Equine Veterinary Science* 34, 1076–1083.

Soroko, M., Jodkowska, E. and Dudek, K. (2015) [Thermography diagnosis in monitoring annual racehorses' training cycle]. *Medycyna Weterynaryjna* 71, 52–58 (in Polish).

Stephan, E. and Gorlach, A. (1971) Measuring of surface temperatures using infrared thermog-raphy in veterinary medicine. Preliminary report. *Deutsche Tierarztliche Wochenschrift* 78, 330–332.

Strömberg, B. (1971) The normal and diseased superficial flexor tendon in racehorses. A morpho-logic and physiologic investigation. *Acta Radiologica Supplementum* 305, 1–94.

Strömberg, B. (1972) Thermography of the superficial flexor tendon in racehorses. *Acta Radiologica Supplementum* 319, 295–297.

Strömberg, B. (1974) The use of thermography in equine orthopedics. *Journal of the American Veterinary Radiology Association* 5, 94–97.

Sullivan, K.A., Hill, A.E. and Haussler, K.K. (2005) The effects of chiropractic, massage and phenylbutazone on spinal mechanical nociceptive thresholds in horses without clinical signs. *Equine Veterinary Journal* 40, 14–20.

Tunley, B.V. and Henson, F.M. (2004) Reliability and repeatability of thermographic examination and the normal thermographic image of the thoracolumbar region in the horse. *Equine Veterinary Journal* 36, 306–312.

Turner, T.A. (1991) Thermography as an aid to the clinical lameness evaluation. *Veterinary Clinics of North America: Equine Practice* 7, 311–338.

Turner, T.A. (1996) Thermography as an aid in the localization of upper hindlimb lameness. *Pferdeheilkunde* 12, 632–634.

Turner, T.A. (1998) The use of thermography in lameness evaluation. *Proceedings of the American Association of Equine Practitioners* 44, 224–226.

Turner, T.A. (2001) Diagnostic thermography. *Veterinary Clinics of North America: Equine Practice* 17, 95–113.

Turner, T.A. (2003) Thermography: use in equine lameness. In: Ross, M.W. and Dyson, S.J. (eds) *Diagnosis and Management of Lameness in the Horse*. Elsevier, St Louis, Missouri.

Turner, T.A. and Scoggins, R.D. (1985) Thermographic detection of gingering in horses. *Journal of Equine Veterinary Science* 5, 8–10.

Turner, T.A., Fessler, J.F., Lamp, M., Pearce, J.A. and Geddes, L.A. (1983) Thermographic evalu-ations of podotrochlosis in horses. *American Journal of Veterinary Research* 44, 535–539.

Turner, T.A., Purohit, R.C. and Fessler, J.F. (1986) Thermography: a review in equine medicine. *Compendium of Continuing Education* 8, 855–861.

Turner, T.A., Rantanen, N.W. and Hauser, M.L. (1996) Alternate methods of soft tissue imaging. The equine athlete: tendon, ligament and soft tissue injuries. In: *Proceedings of the 1996 Dubai International Equine Symposium*, 27–30 March 1996, Dubai, UAE, pp. 165–176.

Turner, T.A., Pansch, J. and Wilson, J.H. (2001) Thermographic assessment of racing Thoroughbreds. *American Association of Equine Practitioners* 47, 344–346.

Vaden, M.F., Purohit, R.C., McCoy, M.D. and Vaughan, J.T. (1980) Thermography: a technique for subclinical diagnosis of osteoarthritis. *American Journal of Veterinary Research* 41, 1175–1179.

Valera, M., Bartolomé, E., Sánchez, M.J., Molina, A., Cook, N.J. and Schaefer, A.L. (2012) Changes in eye temperature and stress assessment in horses during show jumping competitions. *Journal of Equine Veterinary Science* 32, 827–830.

Van Hoogmoed, L.M., Snyder, J.R., Allen, A.K. and Waldsmith, J.D. (2000) Use of infrared thermography to detect performance-enhancing techniques in horses. *Equine Veterinary Education* 12, 102–107.

Verschooten, F., Desmet, P. and Verbeeck, J. (1997) Skin surface temperature measurements in horses by electronic thermometry. *Equine Practice* 19, 16–23.

von Schweinitz, D.G. (1998) Thermographic evidence for the effectiveness of acupuncture in equine neuromuscular disease. *Acupuncture in Medicine* 16, 14–17.

von Schweinitz, D.G. (1999) Thermographic diagnosis in equine back pain. *Veterinary Clinics of North America: Equine Practice* 15, 161–177.

Waldsmith, J.K. and Oltmann, J.I. (1994) Thermography: subclinical inflammation, diagnosis, rehabilitation and athletic evaluation. *Journal of Equine Veterinary Science* 14, 8–10.

Westermann, S., Stanek, C., Schramel, J.P., Ion, A. and Buchner, H.H. (2013) The effect of airflow on thermographically determined temperature of the distal forelimb of the horse. *Equine Veterinary Journal* 45, 637–641.

Last veterinarian visit:	Type of current treatment:	Previous injuries of the musculoskeletal system:
ENVIRONMENTAL CONDITIONS		
Type of examination room:	Ambient temperature:	Outside temperature (if examination takes place indoors):
PREPARATION OF HORSE FOR EXAMINATION		
Length of rest time:	Time to acclimatize:	Characterization of the hair coat:
Type of training on the day and before examination:	Presence of rugs or bandages before examination:	Others:
Any other additional information		

Index